The Anti-Inflammatory Guide
© 2023 Future Publishing Limited

Future Books is an imprint of Future PLC
Quay House, The Ambury, Bath, BA1 1UA

A catalogue record for this book is
available from the British Library.

ISBN 978-1-80521-330-7 hardback

The paper holds full FSC certification
and accreditation.

Printed in Turkey by Ömür Printing, for Future PLC

**Interested in Foreign Rights to publish this title?
Email us at:**
licensing@futurenet.com

Editor
Sarah Bankes

Art Editor
Lora Barnes

Contributors
Julie Bassett, Ailsa Harvey, Sara Niven

Senior Art Editor
Andy Downes

Head of Art & Design
Greg Whitaker

Editorial Director
Jon White

Managing Director
Grainne McKenna

SVP Lifestyle, Knowledge and News
Sophie Wybrew-Bond

Production Project Manager
Matthew Eglinton

Global Business Development Manager
Jennifer Smith

Head of Future International & Bookazines
Tim Mathers

Cover images
Getty Images

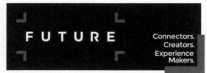

Future plc is a public company
quoted on the London Stock
Exchange
(symbol: FUTR)
www.futureplc.com

Chief Executive Officer **Jon Steinberg**
Non-Executive Chairman **Richard Huntingford**
Chief Financial and Strategy Officer **Penny Ladkin-Brand**

Tel +44 (0)1225 442 244

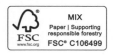

— THE —
ANTI-INFLAMMATORY
Guide

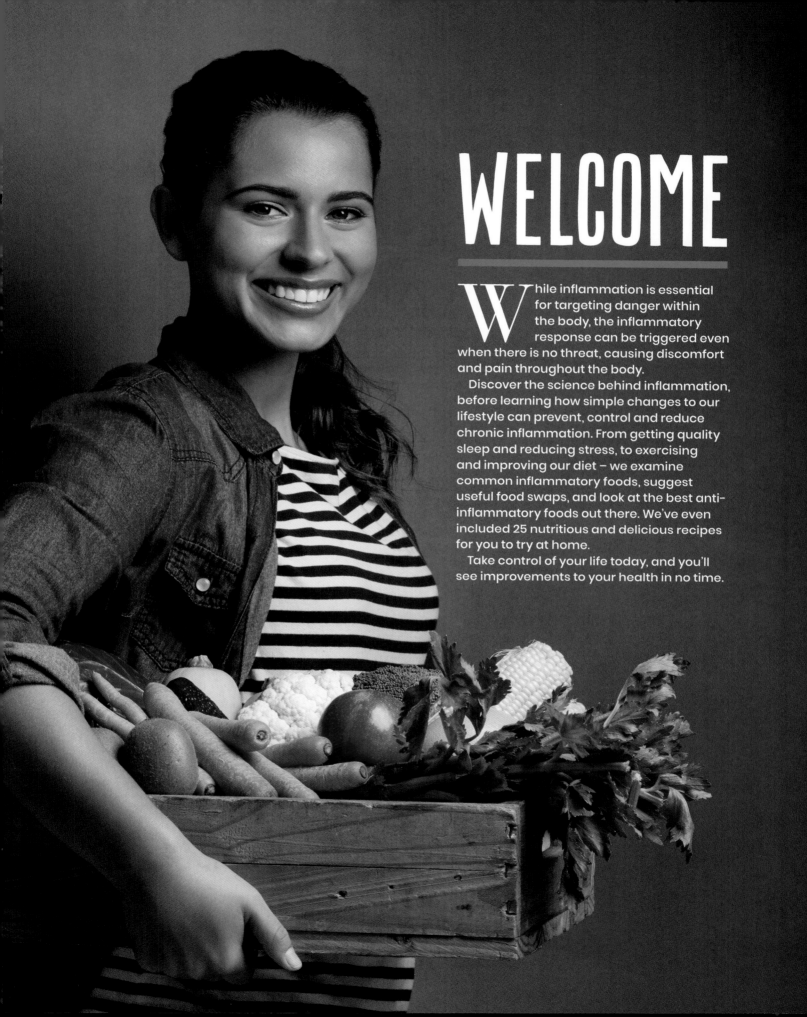

WELCOME

While inflammation is essential for targeting danger within the body, the inflammatory response can be triggered even when there is no threat, causing discomfort and pain throughout the body.

Discover the science behind inflammation, before learning how simple changes to our lifestyle can prevent, control and reduce chronic inflammation. From getting quality sleep and reducing stress, to exercising and improving our diet – we examine common inflammatory foods, suggest useful food swaps, and look at the best anti-inflammatory foods out there. We've even included 25 nutritious and delicious recipes for you to try at home.

Take control of your life today, and you'll see improvements to your health in no time.

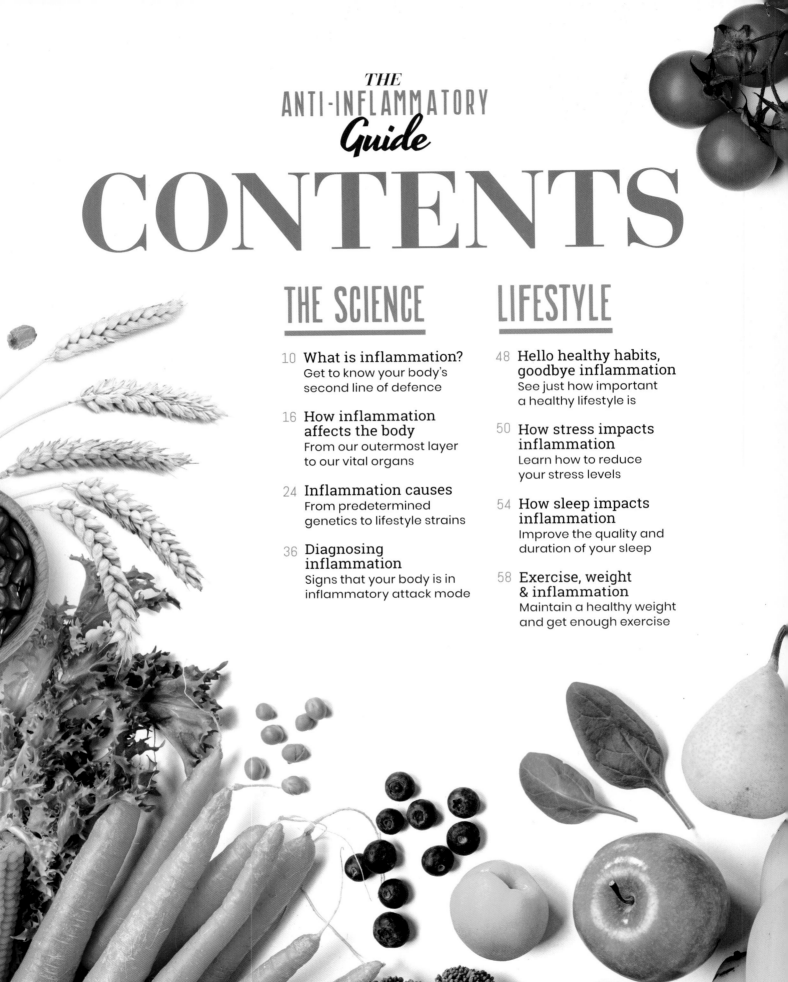

THE ANTI-INFLAMMATORY Guide

CONTENTS

THE SCIENCE

LIFESTYLE

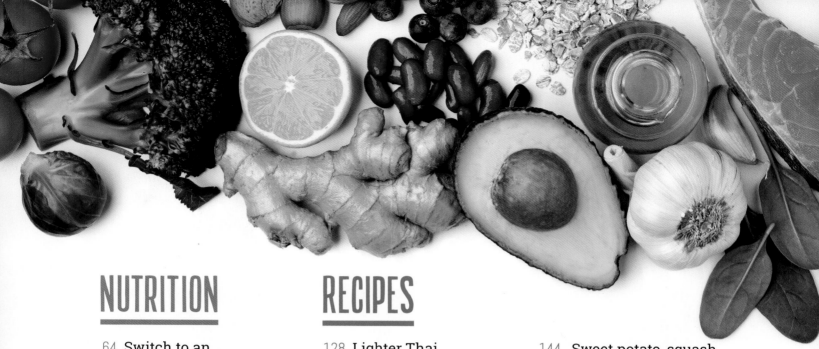

NUTRITION

RECIPES

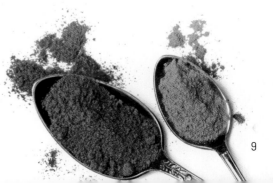

© Getty

WHAT IS
inflammation?

Get to know your body's second line
of defence, including how it can sometimes
cause more harm than good

© Getty

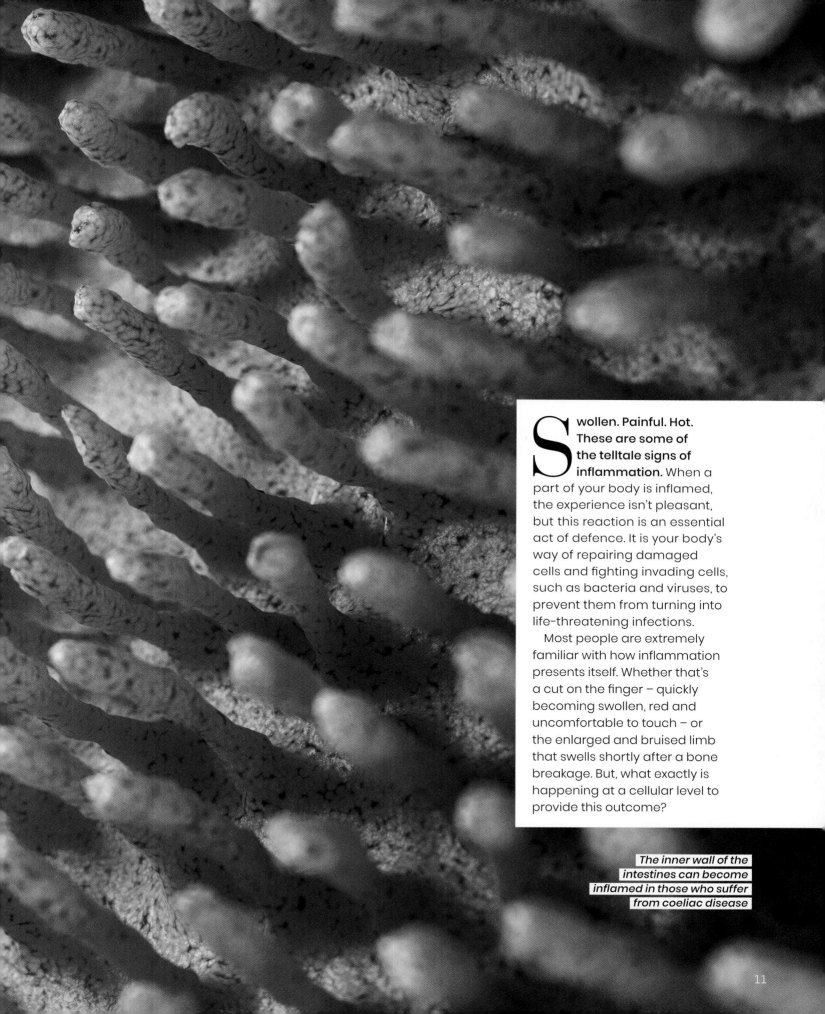

Swollen. Painful. Hot. These are some of the telltale signs of inflammation. When a part of your body is inflamed, the experience isn't pleasant, but this reaction is an essential act of defence. It is your body's way of repairing damaged cells and fighting invading cells, such as bacteria and viruses, to prevent them from turning into life-threatening infections.

Most people are extremely familiar with how inflammation presents itself. Whether that's a cut on the finger – quickly becoming swollen, red and uncomfortable to touch – or the enlarged and bruised limb that swells shortly after a bone breakage. But, what exactly is happening at a cellular level to provide this outcome?

The inner wall of the intestines can become inflamed in those who suffer from coeliac disease

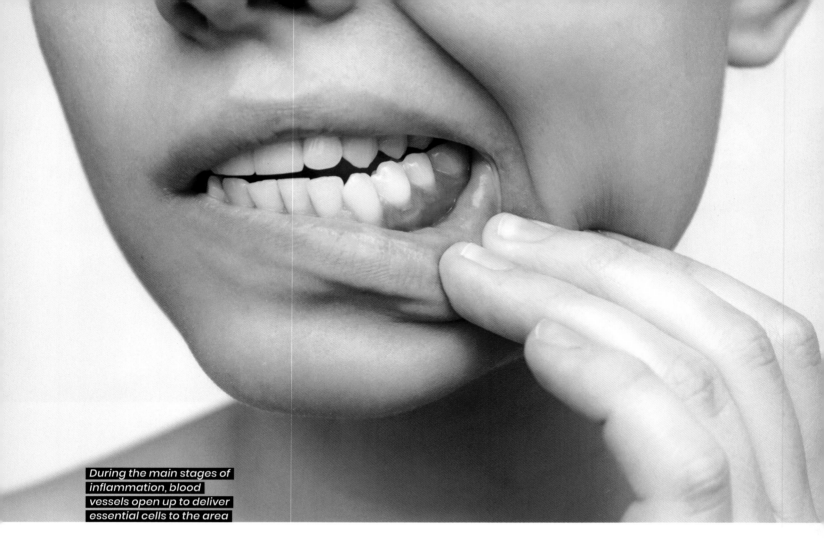

During the main stages of inflammation, blood vessels open up to deliver essential cells to the area

HOW DOES THE BODY CREATE INFLAMMATION?

Inflammation occurs when the body's first protective barriers fail. These barriers include the skin, our largest organ that covers us from head to toe, and the mucus membranes that shield our fragile organs. If harmful, foreign cells find a way through these barriers, they could wreak havoc in our bodies. And that would be the case, if the inflammatory response didn't kick in.

The first stage of the inflammatory response is the inflammatory induction stage, when harmful cells, called pathogens, enter the body. For example, bacteria cells could enter through a cut in the skin and pose a threat to your healthy skin cells. These intruders then begin to attack the body's cells. Each cell comes with unique proteins on their surface, called antigens. When a cell with unrecognisable antigens enters the body, the immune system is triggered, and the first stages of inflammation begins.

Some of the early changes at the site of injury take place in the near blood vessels. First of all, the smaller blood vessels narrow, in order to prevent too much blood from being lost before clotting begins. However, during the main stages of inflammation, these blood vessels need to open up again, to deliver essential cells to the area.

Next, the permeability of their walls increases. This means that instead of limiting the substances that can pass through the walls to just salts and water, more protein can enter the compromised tissue to control the cell invasion.

As some of the cells at the injury site die in the presence of pathogens, they release a warning signal in the form of chemicals. Cells that release these signals are called chemokines. These signals are also released during physical injury caused by skin breakage. Some of the chemicals released are histamine, bradykinin and prostaglandins. The presence of these chemicals alert white blood cells to the danger. These blood cells, called phagocytes,

The acute response
How dying tissue is healed

1.Creating a cut
When an object cuts through your skin, the depth determines how much damage is sustained and how great the inflammatory response needs to be.

2.The skin's surface
The skin makes up 15% of your body weight, and hosts 1.5 trillion bacterial cells.

3.Bacteria beyond the barrier
Wounds provide a gateway for bacteria to enter the body.

4.Signalling cells
The cells that come into contact with dangerous bacteria release chemicals such as histamine.

5.Signal response
In response to the histamine, the blood vessels enlarge to increase the volume of blood cells being pumped to the area.

6.Wound and swelling
Swelling or bruising around the injury begins within half an hour of the skin being pierced.

7.Fleet of phagocytes
Signals called vasodilators loosen the endothelial cells that line the walls of our blood vessels. This makes it easier for phagocytes to pass out of the bloodstream.

8.Phagocyte feast
As the phagocytes engulf pathogens and infected cells, they encourage new, healthy skin cells to be produced.

9.Reduced swelling
The damaged cells become replaced by healthy cells, and the swelling around the wound gradually lessens, until completely healed.

target the area and engulf the bacteria, along with any lingering dead cells.

The quantity of white blood cells depends on the extent of damage. When you sustain a small injury, such as a fly bite, there will be enough white blood cells already circulating in the body to take care of the situation.

More extreme damage, however, requires newly made blood cells to be released. Some of these may not be fully developed yet, but are better than nothing. Due to the need

for a high volume of phagocytes, they are sent out to achieve their purpose as first responders early.

Another reaction that takes place, following the release of the chemical signals, is that the surrounding blood vessels at the area of injury are signalled to release fluid into the tissue around the cut. This creates the puffy appearance that occurs during swelling. The reason for this is to increase the defence around the bacteria or other pathogens. As the tissue volume is filled with fluid, and the

volume of the area increases, it becomes harder for the harmful cells to travel into other areas of the body.

An inflamed cut is often coupled with oozing pus. When you injure yourself, your wounds might weep this clear liquid for the next day or two. This stage of injury is a sign that your body is working hard to protect itself and is in the process of healing. Some of the products of inflammation, including dead bacteria, dead tissue and dead phagocytes, exit the wound in the pus.

THE IMPACT OF FOOD

The chances of developing chronic inflammation isn't always predetermined. One factor that can greatly affect the levels of inflammation in the body is our diet. C-reactive proteins (CRP) are made by the liver, and increase in number during an inflammatory response. While these are made to aid inflammation when needed, their production can also increase in the bloodstreams of people who eat a lot of processed foods. Other foods, such as a selection of fruits and vegetables, have proven to be anti-inflammatory.

One food product that causes significant inflammation, but only in certain people, is gluten. People with coeliac disease, an autoimmune disease, can't eat gluten without their bodies instigating an immune response. This includes problematic inflammation of the intestines that can damage the tiny hair-like structures lining the intestine, essential for optimal absorption of nutrients from food.

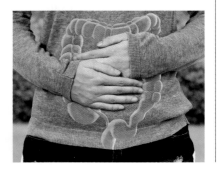

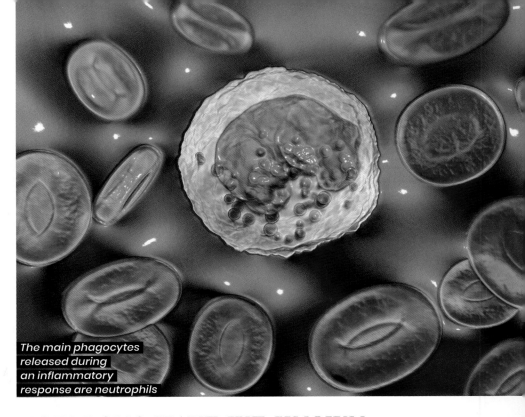

The main phagocytes released during an inflammatory response are neutrophils

HOW LONG HAVE WE KNOWN ABOUT INFLAMMATION?

The earliest understood record of a description for inflammation comes from the first century. A Roman physician, named Celsus, described the biological response as rubor (redness), tumor (swelling), with calor (heat) and dolor (pain).

Before it was known that inflammation was a defence reaction, it was thought to be a disease, due to the pain and swelling it caused. This was until late in the 18th century, when a surgeon from London, named John Hunter, realised that inflammation benefitted the body most of the time, and served instead to prevent disease.

The more detailed knowledge of the inflammatory response, which we have today, is credited to the invention of the compound microscope in the 16th century. As the resolution and quality of this microscope increased over the years, visibility of the movements and details of cells during cases of inflammation improved. Details such as the movement of blood flow and the changes in the composition of inflamed tissue were analysed by such microscopes.

> The word 'inflammation' comes from the Latin word 'inflammare', meaning 'to set on fire'.

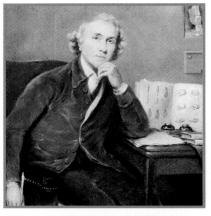

Surgeon John Hunter (inset) held the theory that inflammation was a reaction of the small blood vessels to disease

Acute Chronic

Inflammation is essential for targeting danger within the body, but in some instances the inflammatory response is triggered even when there is no threat to the body. When the reaction occurs solely to remove pathogens from the body, it is known as acute inflammation, whereas chronic inflammation is more detrimental, with more painful symptoms to endure.

When performing properly, the inflammatory system relies on regulatory measures to release the correct doses of defence cells, and causes inflammation only when the body is hurt. If the regulatory mechanism is defected, inflammation can persist for longer than necessary, making the uncomfortable symptoms longer-lasting.

The two terms define how long the symptoms of inflammation last. Most people experience acute inflammation, which only persists for a matter of hours or days. However, chronic inflammation sufferers may experience pain for many months and even years.

Psoriasis presents as raised patches of reddened, thick skin

Commonly, people with chronic inflammation also suffer from cancer, heart disease, diabetes, Alzheimer's or arthritis. The latter causes chronic inflammation that impacts areas surrounding the joints. Those who suffer from rheumatoid arthritis will suffer periodically from significant joint pain, as white blood cells consistently target tissues of the joint.

The effects of chronic inflammation differ depending on the cause and the region of the body impacted. For example, if you suffer from systemic lupus – a condition that causes the immune system to attack its own cells throughout the body – you are likely to suffer from fatigue, as the cells are constantly working harder. Systemic lupus usually targets a variety of cells, such as those in the joints, skin, brain, lungs, kidneys and blood vessels.

Tuberculosis is a disease, caused by bacteria, which can also bring on chronic inflammation. When the bacterium Mycobacterium tuberculosis enters the body, it targets the lungs. As these pathogens attack the cells, it causes feverous symptoms.

Chronic inflammation can produce pain in the abdomen, chest or other internal areas, but it can also irritate the body at

Inflammation of the brain's active tissue is called encephalitis.

Arthritis can make joints painful to move, stiff and warm

surface level. Skin conditions, such as psoriasis, are caused by inflammation of the skin. As the skin is regularly attacked by the immune system, the rate of production of new skin cells is increased in psoriasis sufferers. This produces a rash due to inflammation and itchy skin as new cells are constantly being made. During this build-up of new skin cells, the skin may also appear bumpy.

From the lifesaving cases of inflammation, to these infuriating over-stimulated inflammatory responses, scientists' knowledge of this complex response is growing. Today, there are many medications that can be used to relieve some of the discomfort of acute inflammation, such as aspirin, paracetamol and ibuprofen. With further study, scientists hope to improve the lives of those who suffer from the less well understood, and much more diverse, chronic inflammatory responses, too.

HOW INFLAMMATION *affects the body*

Any part of the body that is susceptible to damage can quickly become an inflammation site

When you envisage inflammation, your mind is likely to first focus on that at the surface of your body. This is where the symptoms are most noticeable. You may feel a raised lump somewhere in your skin soon after a significant impact, or watch as an array of bumps decorate your hand where you mistakenly picked up a stinging nettle – injecting the chemical irritants of their hairs beneath your body's barrier.

But inflammation occurs out of sight, too – and even beyond feeling. The response can target your joints, muscles and even the most vital organs as they fight to keep you alive. The location of inflammation greatly impacts the seriousness of the symptoms. So, how does this reaction impact the function of different body parts, and how do you know when inflammation is taking place far beneath the skin?

When does inflammation cause pain?

Inflammation causes pain when it impacts various nerves around the body. As an impacted tissue fills with fluid and swells, much more space is occupied by

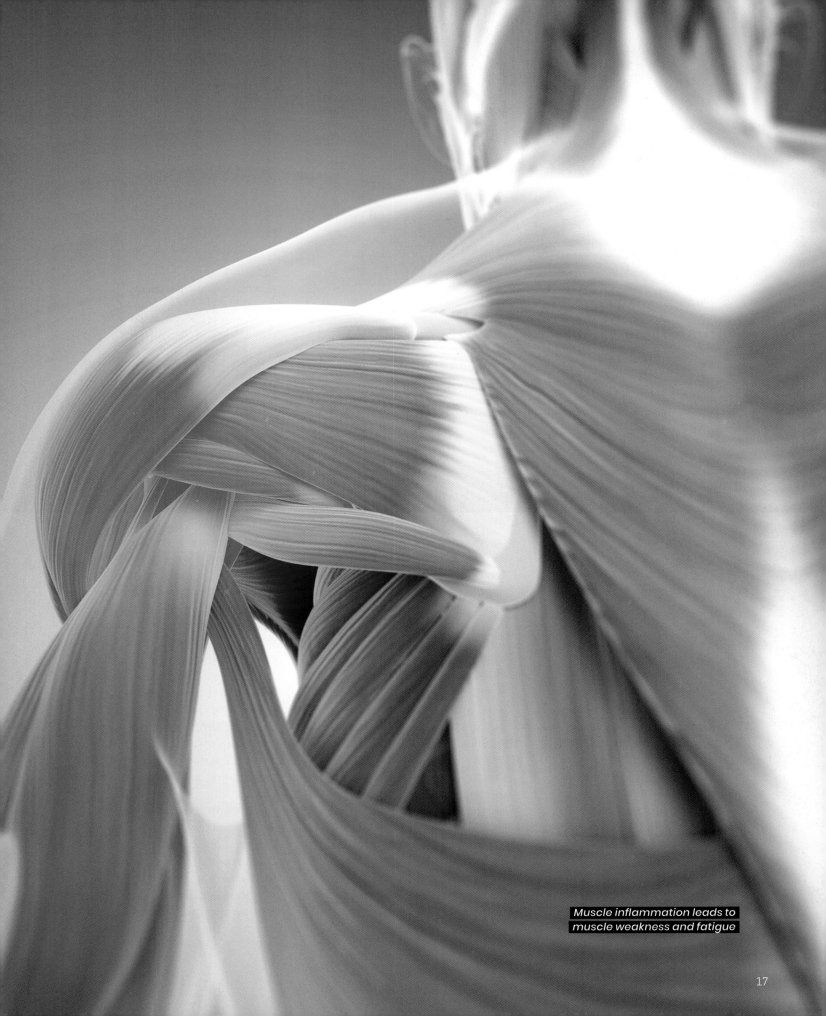

Muscle inflammation leads to muscle weakness and fatigue

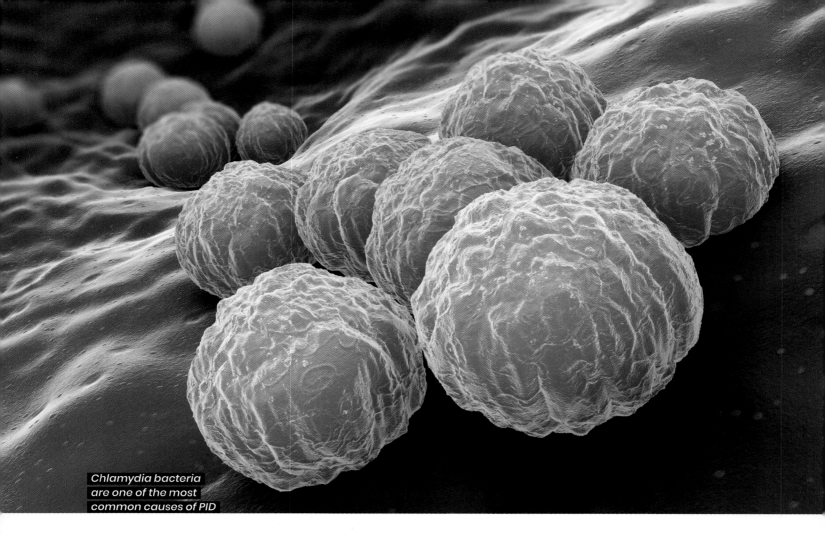

Chlamydia bacteria are one of the most common causes of PID

These swollen tissues press against each other and make contact with sensitive nerve endings. Inflammatory pain can vary throughout the body, and may be relayed as a stabbing, pulsating or pinching sensation.

While some types of chronic inflammation can be excruciating, other forms of inflammation may not transpire into pain. This is because some of our organs don't have as many pain-sensitive nerves. In many instances, this makes chronic inflammation more dangerous, as it can go undetected for longer. For example, it's possible to have an inflamed brain, liver or spleen without feeling any symptoms at all.

Oftentimes, discomfort is only felt in these areas of the body due to inflammation of the tissue surrounding them. The organs with the least pain receptors are solid, while hollow organs usually contain the most. These include the intestines, bladder and uterus.

Minimising muscle strength

Muscles are essential for turning our heads, lifting our legs to walk, arching our backs to sit, or moving the body in any other way. When this tissue becomes inflamed, it is called myositis. Myositis particularly affects the shoulders, hips and thighs, but can limit the function of many other muscles. Muscle inflammation can be brought on by a variety of causes, such as injury, infection and autoimmune disease, resulting in weak, painful and swollen muscles. The most severe myositis conditions are dermatomyositis and polymyositis. Polymyositis is most common in people between the ages of 50 and 70. In some instances, it's triggered by a virus, and mostly involves the inflammation of muscles closest to the trunk of the body. The cause of dermatomyositis is unknown, but has similar features to an autoimmune disease, with the added symptom of a skin rash.

In contrast to these long-term conditions, injury-induced inflammation in muscles can result from vigorous exercise. In these instances, muscles are weakened for hours or days after exercise and are repaired following rest.

Pathogens are also capable of reaching the muscles and infecting them, bringing on inflammation. A variety of pathogen types can cause this, but by far the most common are viruses. These enter muscle tissue directly, or cause damage to muscle fibres by releasing toxic substances in the surrounding tissue. The types of virus that can inflame muscles vary and include the widespread common cold. Muscle tissue is usually highly resistant to pathogen invasion, but during injury they become more susceptible to infection.

Symptoms in the skin

Being the first point of contact for any substance outside the body, the skin commonly suffers from inflammation from a variety of sources. The most common appearances of inflammation in the skin include rashes, darker pigmentation and blistering. The change in colour – usually red or purple – happens when blood rushes to the impacted area, carrying cells for healing. Blood vessels widen to bring blood closer to the surface.

If your skin has ever broken out in blotchy, raised bumps, you have suffered from an inflammatory reaction. There are numerous skin conditions, characterised by inflammatory reactions. One such

Including green, leafy vegetables in your diet is one way to reduce inflammation in the body.

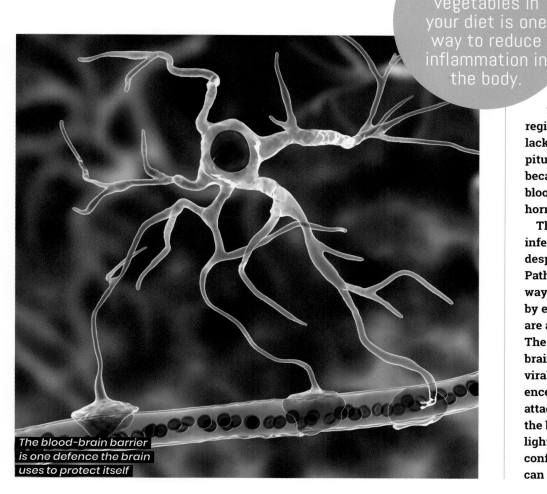

The blood-brain barrier is one defence the brain uses to protect itself

BREAKING THE BLOOD-BRAIN BARRIER

Your brain is arguably the most important organ in which to prevent inflammation and damage, due to its high level of control over the rest of the body. Because of this function, the organ has evolved to be the most physically protected. Its full defence package includes a skull casing, multiple membranes and a layer of protective fluid. The latter is called the blood-brain barrier (BBB).

Located between the brain and the bloodstream, this layer restricts which substances can enter the brain to prevent the likes of pathogens and toxins from infecting it. Some regions of the brain, however, lack this barrier. The posterior pituitary is one of these areas, because it needs access to the bloodstream to directly release hormones that are made there.

The brain still suffers from infection and inflammation, despite the blood-brain barrier. Pathogens have found some ways to cross over, such as by entering other cells that are allowed to pass through. The most common cause of brain inflammation is due to viral infection, called viral encephalitis. As viruses attack brain cells, causing the brain to swell, headaches, light sensitivity, a stiff neck, confusion or memory loss can ensue.

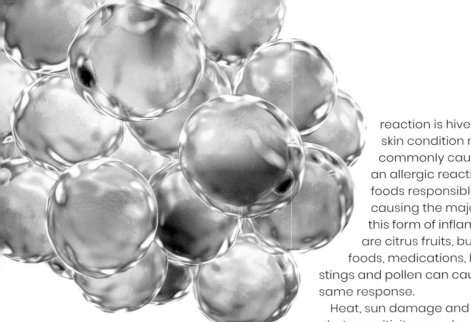

HOW DOES OBESITY INFLUENCE INFLAMMATION?

Research shows that some of the conditions that cause the immune system to consistently attack parts of the body – leading to ongoing inflammation – is linked to obesity. When people are overweight, the fat cells can act as if they are under pathogenic attack, causing the body's immune cells to enter the fatty tissue and increase inflammation.

As the level of chronic inflammation increases with weight gain, this also causes the fat cells to release more of the hormone leptin. When leptin levels reach high levels, the body's energy balance is altered, making a person feel hungry more often – even when they don't require more energy.

Leptin contributes to chronic inflammation and creates a detrimental cycle. As the hormone encourages an already overweight person to keep eating, fat cells accumulate to contribute to inflammation and the further production of leptin.

reaction is hives, a skin condition most commonly caused by an allergic reaction. The foods responsible for causing the majority of this form of inflammation are citrus fruits, but other foods, medications, bites, stings and pollen can cause the same response.

Heat, sun damage and photosensitivity can also make the skin inflamed. A heat rash is a result of the skin's sweat glands becoming blocked. When this happens, sweat can't reach the skin's surface to evaporate and becomes trapped. This may result in blisters forming, or itchy and inflamed lumps. Heat rashes can be caused by exposure to the sun – and the power of the sky's fireball doesn't end there.

Photosensitivity, also known as an allergic reaction to the sun, is an immune reaction to sunlight. Signs that you are allergic to the sun include becoming covered in inflamed, red patches or a series of bumps over your skin once it has been exposed to sunlight. Many light-skinned people turn red when burnt by UV radiation, but photosensitivity is an inflammatory reaction to the light itself, distinguishable by its patchy pattern.

Seeing threats
Your eyes are relatively fragile organs. But they're not immune to inflammation. Uveitis is the term used to describe all types

of optical inflammation. In some instances this is acute inflammation, but chronic inflammation poses a greater risk of vision impairment.

Different parts of the eye can be subject to inflammation. Conjunctivitis is a condition that causes inflammation of the eyeball's mucus membrane, keratitis is that of the cornea – the clear, dome-shaped lens covering the front of the eye – and thyroid eye disease (TED) targets the muscle and fat behind the eyeball. If you suspect any inflammation of the eye, the best option is to see a medical expert as soon as you can. Most of the time, these can be treated with few after-effects, but when left untreated for too long, inflammation can begin to impede vision.

Does inflammation get on your nerves?
When a single nerve, or a group, becomes inflamed it is called neuritis. These fibre bundles serve as messengers between the body and brain. Designed to pick up the smallest pieces of information, it's no wonder that nerve inflammation is capable of causing intense pain.

Sensory neuron inflammation is experienced as burning and stabbing pains, while motor neuron inflammation causes muscle weakness. This is because the role of sensory neurons is to relay information about changes in the environment, while motor

> **High levels of inflammation in the brain has been linked to depression.**

© Getty

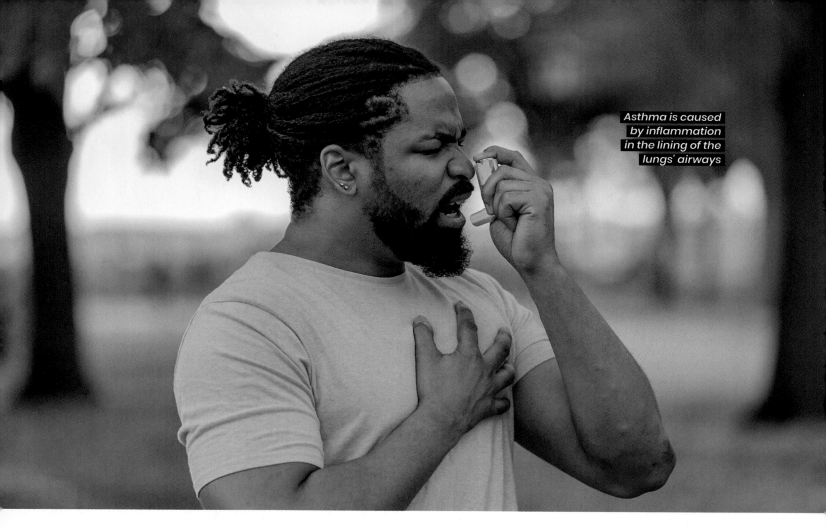

neurons link the brain and body in order to move muscles when we want or need to. A sensory neuron needs to keep signals firing to the brain at every slight change in sensation – a trait that becomes lifesaving when the body is in contact with a boiling-hot object, causing the body to retreat. When inflamed, these nerve cells are overstimulated and regularly firing pain signals.

Inflamed breathing

Our lungs are giant sacs that are constantly cycling life-sustaining air. To function in this way, the air needs to be able to enter the lungs easily. Without any thought, we draw oxygen into our lungs, releasing waste gas each time. Unfortunately, this passage to the centre of one of our most vital organs, can also be a route taken by dangerous pathogens.

When airborne irritants enter the lungs, they impair the many tiny sacs lining the lungs' surfaces. As these become inflamed, oxygen struggles to pass through them, making breathing far more difficult. If lung inflammation is left untreated for too long, the air sacs lose their flexibility over time, stopping them from expanding with each breath, as they are supposed to.

How does inflammation impair filtration?

The kidneys work together to serve as your body's filtration system. Inflammation of these organs can impact just one or both at the same time. When both kidneys become inflamed, this is most detrimental, because it is possible to have one damaged one removed and still live a healthy life.

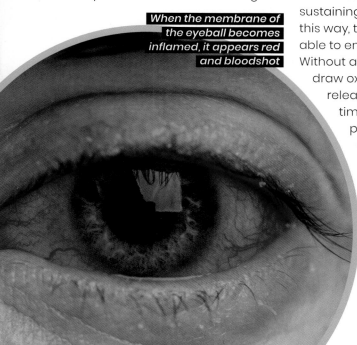

When the membrane of the eyeball becomes inflamed, it appears red and bloodshot

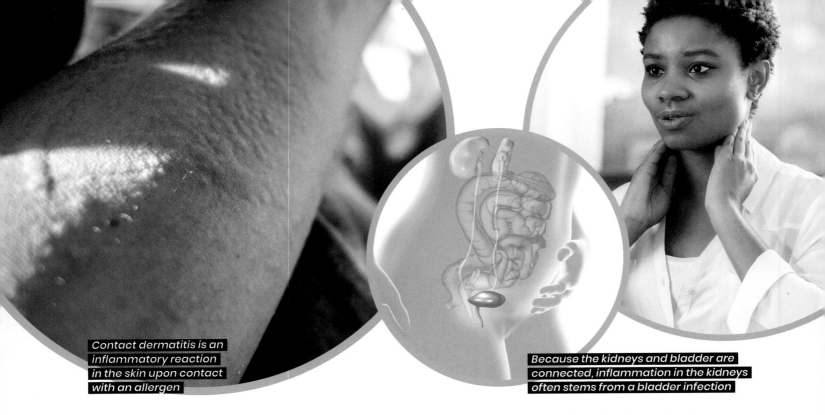

Contact dermatitis is an inflammatory reaction in the skin upon contact with an allergen

Because the kidneys and bladder are connected, inflammation in the kidneys often stems from a bladder infection

A pair of healthy kidneys filters 200 litres of fluid, removing toxins from the blood to be released in the urine. If they become inflamed, their tubes can become swollen, limiting how much liquid can pass through, or the tiny blood capillaries can be targeted. If blood can't pass through all the capillaries, the kidneys are unable to filter toxins optimally.

This form of inflammation can begin as a bacterial infection in the bladder, which travels into the kidneys. Some signs that you could be suffering from kidney inflammation are abdominal or pelvic pains, an increased urge to urinate and high blood pressure.

Why are glands prone to swelling?

Have you ever felt your neck or armpit when suffering from a cold, to find an unfamiliar lump? This is a result of swollen lymph nodes, caused by the presence of a bacterium or virus. These clusters of cells are called glands, and they span your entire body, specifically tasked with trapping infections before they spread further. During a pathogen invasion, inflammation is most common in the neck, under the chin and armpits, and in the groin. When white blood cells are signalled to kill pathogens, they are usually summoned to lymph nodes.

The inflammation of other glands can have more serious consequences, however. The thyroid gland, which is located in the neck, is responsible for regulating the speed of your body's cell activity. The use of some medications, radiation exposure or autoimmune diseases are some of the causes of thyroid inflammation.

Human breast milk contains anti-inflammatory proteins.

When the thyroid is inflamed, pain is felt in the neck, jaw and ears. As the thyroid becomes swollen, the change in tissue can either result in the thyroid hormone being trapped – and not entering the blood – or too high a quantity leaking into the bloodstream. Usually, this hormone regulates the rate at which your food is broken down in the body to produce energy. Uncontrolled quantities in the blood can become dangerous quickly. Too much of it can cause rapid weight loss and an irregular heartbeat, and too little can knock someone unconscious.

The dangers of having a big heart

Unlike the metaphor, literally having a big heart does not make someone better, but can cause serious issues. We rely on our beating hearts to provide a constant circulation of essential nutrients to every part of our bodies. Any inflammation of this vital organ can greatly impact this blood flow.

When infection or injury reaches the heart, its valves, lining, muscle or the tissue surrounding it become inflamed. In cases where the muscle is inflamed, the crucial pumping motions are impacted, along with the volume of blood that circulates. This condition is called myocarditis and can leave you with chest pain and shortness of breath, and create an irregular heart rhythm. These are serious symptoms and, if they are not checked and treated, there is an increased risk of clotting and a heart attack.

A viral infection is the most common cause of myocarditis, but many people develop an inflamed heart obliviously. Oftentimes, no symptoms arise due to a slight inflammation. If your doctor detects signs of myocarditis, you might be told to reduce exercise as a precaution and be recommended a low-salt diet. This helps to reduce any fluid build-up in your heart.

What is pelvic inflammatory disease (PID)?

The female reproductive system comprises internal and external organs – many of which can become affected by inflammation. Grouped under one term, pelvic inflammatory disease (PID) describes the infection of any female reproductive organ, such as the vagina, uterus and ovaries.

The most common cause of inflammation from PID is a bacterial infection of gonorrhoea or chlamydia. These usually enter the body during unprotected sex and cause inflammation of the upper genital tract. Sometimes this inflammation causes no symptoms, while in other instances it causes significant pain in the lower abdomen. In men, too, these pathogens infect the gential tract and can cause swelling in the testicles.

Bacterial infections are one of the most common forms of infertility in men and women, and any discomfort should be checked out. Regular testing and seeking treatment can help to eliminate infection and prevent inflammation from damaging reproductive organs.

IMPACT-INDUCED INFLAMMATION

Instantly sustained cuts and bites are commonly associated with injury-induced inflammation. However, a repetitive action, such as the impact of your leg hitting the ground while running, can cause the eventual inflammation of joints.

Muscle tears, injured tendons, 'tennis elbow' and 'runner's knee' are some of the most common causes of inflammation due to sport. Your rotator cuff is a group of muscles surrounding your shoulder joints that connect your shoulder to your upper arm. When someone repeats the movement of lifting their arm over their head, (for example, when swinging a racket) these muscles can tear. The swelling that results from the inflammation around these muscles limits movement in the shoulder joint until the tissue is repaired.

Runner's knee – technically called patellofemoral pain syndrome – is caused by irritation under the kneecap, from the continuous impact of running or jumping. Inflammation arises where the front of the knee connects to the thigh bone. Tennis elbow (lateral epicondylitis) is inflammation of the elbow that occurs when the tendons are overused. The common name for this condition is due to the many instances of lateral epicondylitis among tennis players after the strenuous wrist movements required in training.

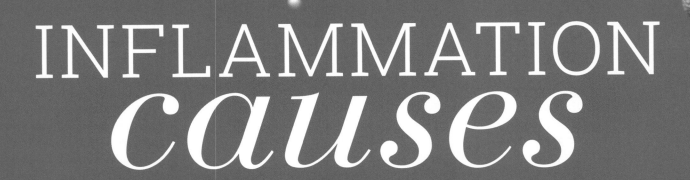

INFLAMMATION *causes*

From predetermined genetics to lifestyle strains, what factors put our bodies in extreme defence mode?

Inflammation is one word – one term to categorise numerous autoimmune diseases, allergies and injuries, capable of producing a multitude of different reactions throughout the body. While all of the core responses are the same in inflammation, the reactions in the body and the root causes greatly vary. One of the main causes of inflammation is infection due to the entrance of pathogens into the body, and the biggest cause of chronic inflammation comes from leaving some of these infections untreated. As blood flow increases in infected tissue, immune cells are delivered to the foreign cells. What follows is a battle of blood cells versus pathogens. If the immune response fails to eliminate all the harmful cells, it's possible for infection to linger in the body for extended periods – becoming chronic inflammation.

Of course, for some people, it isn't as simple as eliminating the

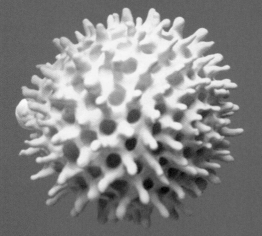

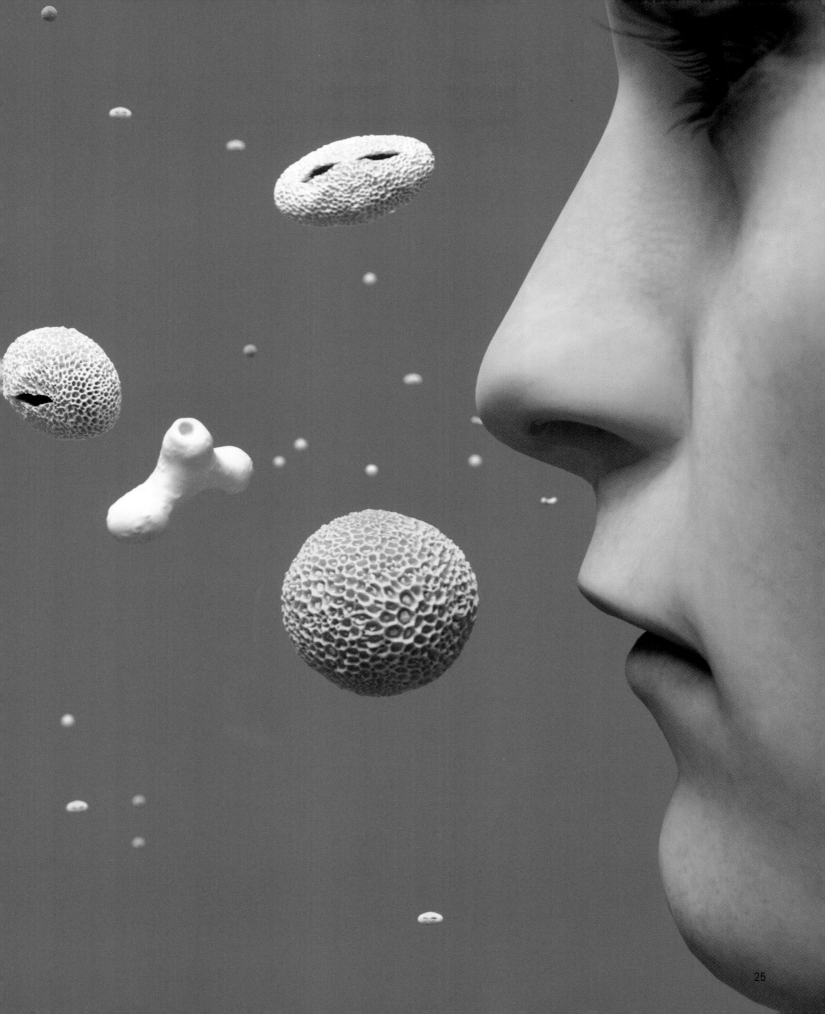

> ## An insect usually deposits saliva into the skin as it inserts its mouthpiece, causing the tissue to become red and itchy

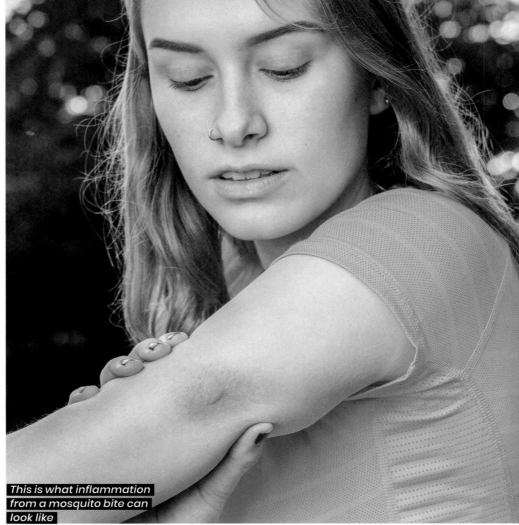

This is what inflammation from a mosquito bite can look like

threat. Chronic inflammatory diseases, which are the body's overreactive response, can arise from the body producing inflammation when there is no threat. Collectively, these diseases are deemed the most significant cause of death by the World Health Organization (WHO). Unfortunately, the number of people living with these diseases, including a variety of autoimmune diseases, is on the rise. Across the world, today around three in five people die as a result of inflammation – mainly respiratory and heart diseases or strokes. From the most serious causes of chronic inflammation, to some of the lifestyle factors that play a small part in

Ticks bury their heads into human skin

maintaining inflammation, knowing the contributors to this painful response can result in a more pain-free life.

The damage of long-term toxin exposure

Toxins are any substance created by animals, plants or microorganisms that are poisonous to humans. There are many ways that these unwanted substances can make their way into the body. This includes being inhaled. Some toxins travel in the air through air passages into the nose and mouth. Others are ingested with food into the stomach and absorbed into the bloodstream. The level of exposure to

different toxins determines the subsequent detriment and inflammation levels. When toxins are being targeted as part of the anti-inflammatory response, the body uses its storage of antioxidants. However, this supply isn't infinite. Prolonged exposure to toxins – whether they be pesticides and other chemicals in the air or heavy metals that have infiltrated drinking water – might cause the body to run low on the molecules needed to keep attacking the harmful cells. If this happens, the body gets run down and inflammation begins to take over. This causes increased pain and ill health.

What's in an insect bite?

Although an insect cuts the skin, the injury itself is too small to

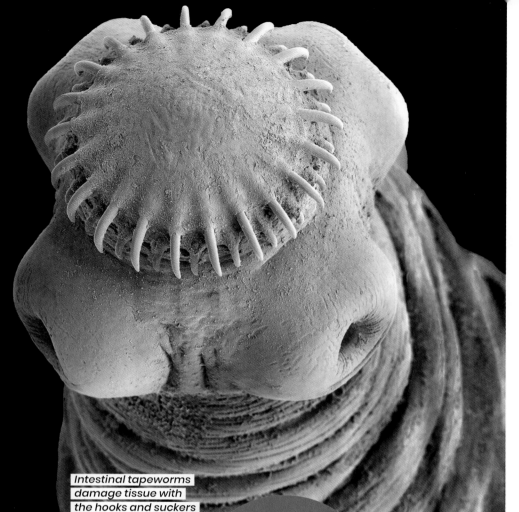

Intestinal tapeworms damage tissue with the hooks and suckers on their heads

Tapeworms can enter the brain and cause an inflammatory reaction.

cause too much inflammatory damage. So then, how can an insect bite result in such an irritating and swollen lump? The cause of this is what enters the body after the bite. An insect usually deposits saliva into the skin as it inserts its mouthpiece, causing the tissue to become red and itchy. In some cases, an insect will inject venom, which can result in a more painful swelling of the skin.

When bacteria enters the insect-made passage into the body, cellulitis can arise. The bacteria, which usually lives relatively un-problematically on the surface of the skin, grows inside the tissue to cause

infection. Scratching at itchy bites can cause the wound to open up further, increasing the risk of infection and inflammation. This is especially true when scratching with dirty fingernails, introducing further pathogens into the body tissue.

The parasites living among us

Some of the insects that cause inflammation are parasites, but not all parasites are insects. A parasite can be any living organism that survives in or on another host. Unfortunately for people, many parasites thrive off many different parts of the human body, depending on what nutrients they seek.

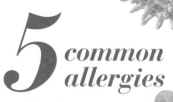

5 common allergies

Hay fever
Allergies to pollen can cause inflammation of the throat, nose, eyes and sinuses. In this process, excessive fluid is produced in the eyes and nose to flush out the allergen.

Dust mites
These mites eat the dead skin cells of all people, but only in those who are allergic to them does an inflammatory response take place. Most often this is presented in the form of itchy skin, nose, eyes and throat.

Food
Inflammation of the lips, tongue and throat can occur immediately after eating food allergens. The most common food allergies are peanuts, milk, eggs, tree nuts and fish.

Latex
Latex is a natural rubber that contains proteins from tree sap. In those with a latex allergy, skin contact with this material causes the skin to become inflamed and break out in a rash.

Mould
A condition called hypersensitivity pneumonitis is caused by an allergic reaction to mould. When breathed in, mould spores trigger an inflammatory response in the lungs.

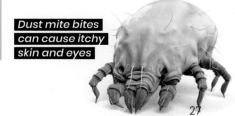

Dust mite bites can cause itchy skin and eyes

How do you know if there is a parasite living off you? In some cases, it is almost impossible to detect their presence, because in order to help them survive they release a numbing agent. A tick – an insect that attaches to the skin and feeds on human blood – is one parasite that does this. While they cause inflammation by leaving swelling under the skin, this may only be felt after the tick has gained all the nutrients it needs.

There are three main types of parasite that, when infecting, can create inflammation in various parts of the body. These are called protozoa, helminth and ectoparasites. Protozoa are single-celled organisms. Protozoan parasites can cause an inflammatory response in the body, if it is able to enter – most commonly in our food and drink.

When inside the body, it invades our healthy cells and relies on them for food and protection. As the foreign cells are detected in the body, inflammation follows. The more advanced single-celled parasites have evolved ways to protect themselves from the immune response, and this can be injurious for the human body. Not only do the parasites remain in the cells for longer, but the longer that the inflammatory response continues for, without success, the more harm it does to healthy human cells.

Helminth are much larger, multicellular parasites, called parasitic worms. These enter the body when ingested, or through bare skin and attach themselves to internal tissues. Often, parasitic worms are found living in the intestines, after hooking themselves onto intestinal walls. When the body recognises the presence of these worms, the intestines become inflamed and irritated. Abdominal pain, swelling and weight loss are all symptoms of helminth infection and inflammation.

The third form of parasite is the ectoparasite, which includes the tick. Instead of attacking

> Pathogen invasion, injury and chemical reactions are the main causes of inflammation.

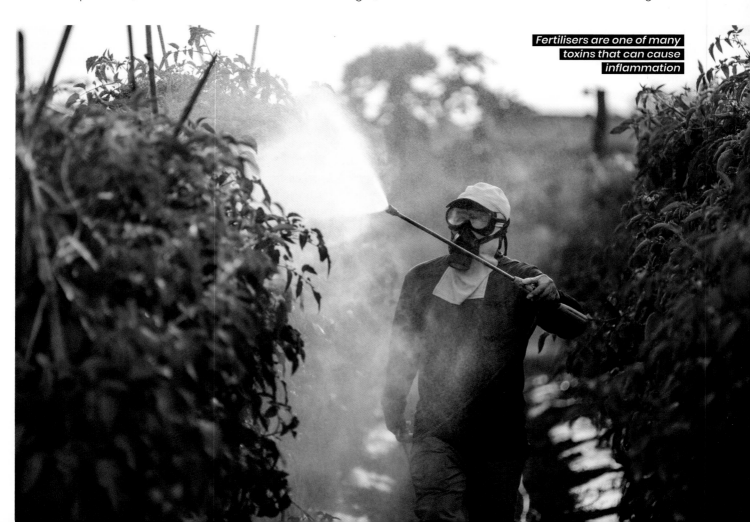

Fertilisers are one of many toxins that can cause inflammation

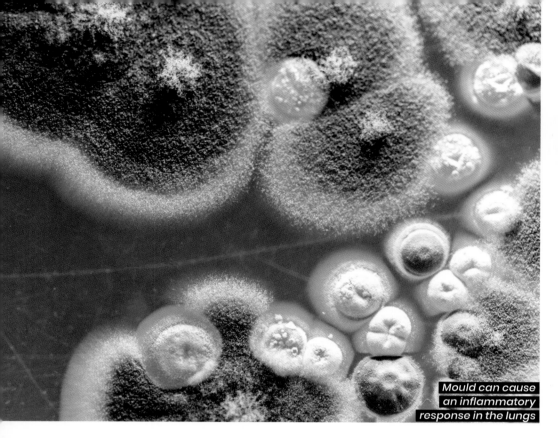

Mould can cause an inflammatory response in the lungs

from the inside, these simply pierce your skin and hope you don't notice while they suck up plentiful nutrients from your blood. Some examples of ectoparasites are lice, mites and bedbugs – and they can remain attached to humans for multiple days at a time.

If you notice another creature stealing your blood, your most instinctual reaction is to speedily remove it from your skin. For some ectoparasite cases, this is the biggest cause of inflammation, as the force used to remove it ruptures the parasite. Any pathogens inside it will then enter the cut skin and cause infection.

What foods ignite an inflammatory battle?

What you eat can greatly influence the levels of inflammation in your body. Some of the main culprits include processed meats, artificial trans fats, oils, sugary foods, refined

> ## " Some of the main culprits include processed meats, oils, sugary foods, refined carbs and excessive alcohol

carbohydrates and excessive alcohol.

The difference between processed and unprocessed meat is that processed meat contains higher levels of advanced glycation end products (AGEs). AGEs are harmful compounds that usually form in the bloodstream when protein and fat is combined with sugar. During the production of processed meat, however, and other foods that have been exposed to high temperatures, this compound is made

ANTI-INFLAMMATORY DRUGS: THE OPPOSITE EFFECT

When suffering from the painful symptoms of inflammation, there aremultiple choices of anti-inflammatory medication you can use to feel more comfortable. But sometimes these drugs rebel and react with the body to instigate further inflammation. There are many reasons for such a reaction, which is why it is important to read the information booklet that comes with the medication. This will explain how to take the medicine and what to do if there are any adverse reactions.

Non-steroidal anti-inflammatory drugs (NSAIDs), such as ibuprofen and aspirin, are produced to tackle inflammation, pain and fever. Because at least one of these symptoms is present in the majority of ailments, NSAIDs are some of the most widely prescribed drugs in the world.

NSAIDs prevent the enzymes responsible for pain and inflammation from working, and these are usually either in the stomach and kidney, or surrounding the joints. Some NSAIDs aren't specific, and target all these enzymes. This means that, while the pain-causing perpetrators will be stopped, so will areas of the body with no inflammation. When overused, these drugs can irritate and inflame the previously healthy areas.

Inflammatory diseases, such as rheumatoid arthritis (the long-term inflammation, pain and stiffness of the joints) can be caused or exacerbated by smoking and drinking. These relatively popular, yet unhealthy, lifestyle habits place the heart and lungs at risk of inflammation and failure.

The tobacco in cigarettes contains unstable electrons called free radicals. When these enter the body, they damage surrounding cells and cause inflammation as part of the healing process. By smoking, you also increase the levels of proteins called cytokines. These proteins are the molecules that attack joints and organs in rheumatoid arthritis sufferers. Meanwhile, drinking too much alcohol can be a driving or additional factor for inflammation of the stomach and liver.

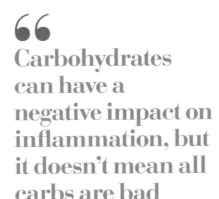

> ❝ Carbohydrates can have a negative impact on inflammation, but it doesn't mean all carbs are bad

before the food is eaten.

When AGEs are made naturally in the body, the levels are relatively low and the body can work to remove them without you noticing. If high volumes of processed meat are eaten, the body is overwhelmed with AGEs and the battle against them is presented as inflammation.

Just as the meat becomes more likely to cause inflammation when it is processed, trans fats are inflammation hazards when they are artificial. Trans fat is the name given to the fat found in animal and dairy products. This is naturally produced when bacteria in an animal's stomach works to digest plants such as grass. At room temperature, trans fats are usually in liquid form. Sometimes, however, these fats are adapted during food production in order to keep them solid at room temperature. When this happens, they have a longer

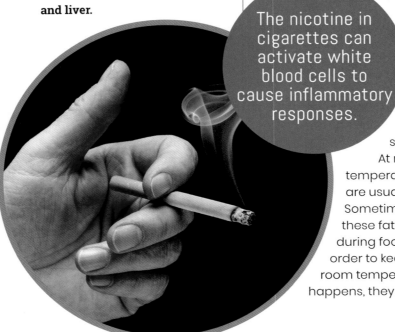

The nicotine in cigarettes can activate white blood cells to cause inflammatory responses.

shelf life and are called artificial trans fats. Although a longer shelf life is good for suppliers, this adaptation comes at a cost to your health.

Multiple studies have shown that increasing these fats in the diet results in a higher number of inflammatory markers being present in the blood. Inflammatory markers is the term given to a group of proteins that are released into the blood when an inflammatory response is triggered.

Some people take no notice during day-to-day life of the fineprint of their blood and other cells, while others try to monitor the levels of different vitamins and minerals in their bodies on a daily basis through supplements. Some nutrients, such as omega-6, have proved to aid various biological functions. Omega-6, which can protect the heart from disease when consumed in moderation, is also an inflammation threat.

This nutrient rarely needs to be added as a supplement, especially in many Western diets, because large numbers of food products provide more omega-6 than a person needs. Vegetable oils contain high concentrations of omega-6, and so foods with great amounts of this oil can cause inflammation to peak. One of the best ways to cancel out some of the negative impacts of vegetable oils is to introduce omega-3 into the diet. Omega-3 is an anti-inflammatory.

Those who don't guide their diet based on nutrient content are likely to choose foods primarily for taste preference – and sugary foods can seem like

© Getty

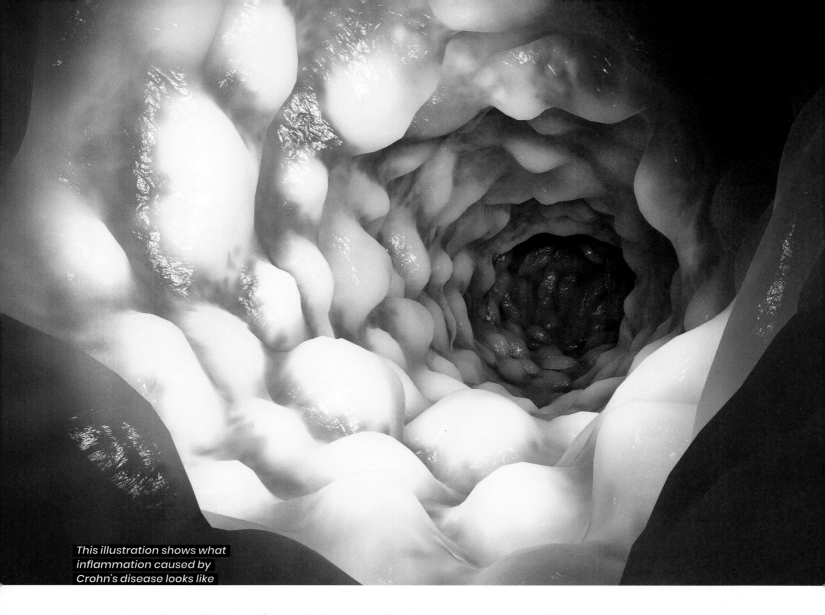

This illustration shows what inflammation caused by Crohn's disease looks like

the perfect feel-good food due to a chemical called serotonin that they release. However, too much sugar can contribute to inflammation, as it stimulates the liver to produce free fatty acids. These are the fatty acids produced when body

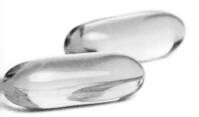

Anti-inflammatory omega-3 supplements can be swallowed in capsules

fat is metabolised. As these are broken down further in the body, they release more harmful compounds, which trigger an inflammatory response.

Carbohydrates can have a negative impact on inflammation, but this doesn't mean all carbohydrates are bad. Only refined carbohydrates are the cause of inflammation flare ups, due to all the nutrients that can be found in most carbohydrates being removed. Fibre is one of these essential nutrients, which is often missing from refined carbohydrates and is responsible for maintaining healthy bacteria in the gut.

When your microbiome – the collection of microorganisms in and on your body – is compromised and includes more of the detrimental bacteria, the immune response is more likely to be launched. Refined carbohydrates often cause inflammatory bacteria to begin growing in the gut, increasing the chances of developing inflammation of the bowel.

For people who suffer from ulcerative colitis or Crohn's disease, limiting their intake of refined carbohydrates can help to manage the symptoms of inflammatory bowel diseases. This, of course, isn't a cure but

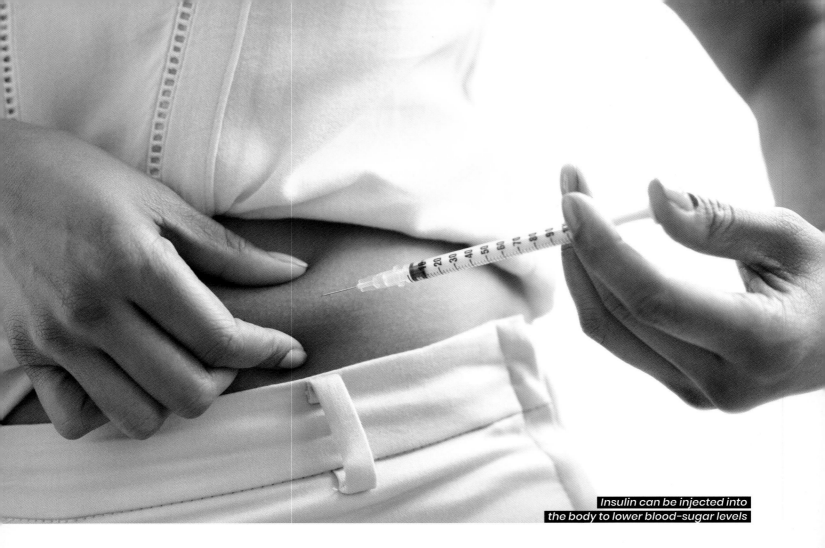

Insulin can be injected into the body to lower blood-sugar levels

demonstrates how analysing and changing what we eat can greatly impact quality of life.

Anti-inflammatory foods

While looking at which foods cause inflammation, and what to avoid, it is worth knowing that there are also foods that can actively reduce it. As mentioned, omega-3 can cancel out some of the inflammation caused by omega-6 fats. This can be found in fatty fish like salmon, sardines and mackerel.

Most anti-inflammatory foods, however, are fruits and vegetables. For example, berries are high in vitamins, minerals and fibre that reduce the likelihood of developing an inflammatory disease. Eating blueberries, in particular, causes the body to produce more immune cells to attack pathogens. This strengthens the inflammatory response to make it a speedier process.

The antioxidants sulforaphane in broccoli, quercetin in bell peppers, phenols in mushrooms, and resveratrol in grapes are just some of many that assist our bodies and stop unwanted inflammation. The antioxidant in grapes has been shown in studies to specifically guard the heart from inflammation.

> Around 7% of the United States population have an intolerance to gluten.

The issue with insulin

Scientists have long been aware that diabetes sufferers are more likely to endure heightened inflammation in the body. But why is this?

If you suffer from diabetes, this means that your blood-sugar level is higher than average. Usually, the hormone insulin works in the body to regulate blood-sugar levels, but a diabetic body shows insulin resistance. The muscle, liver and fat cells fail to respond to insulin, and blood-sugar levels remain high. Instead of being stored in these cells and used as energy, glucose continues to be transported around the body by the blood.

As with most other causes of inflammation, the first step

in launching an inflammatory response comes from the body functioning differently to how it should. In this case, the high levels of glucose produce a threat in the body, and this can occur in a number of ways.

First, the cells that line your blood vessels – called endothelial cells – can be impacted. These are some of the first cells to come into contact with high glucose levels, and they begin to produce reactive molecules called free radicals. This causes an imbalance ratio of free radicals to antioxidants, which is known as oxidative stress. Oxidative stress damages the endothelial cells and, in diabetics, causes chronic inflammation as the cells constantly operate to repair this.

Insulin resistance can also lead to weight gain, caused by the circulating excess sugar. When too much additional fat tissue forms around the waist, and other areas, immune cells are activated. The fat cells release large amounts of inflammation-causing chemicals too.

Can stress cause inflammation?

Do you regularly feel stressed? Perhaps the most noticeable impact this has on your life are the mental factors as you overthink and worry, but at a cellular level this stress can also reduce your body's biological functions. In the most extreme cases of stress, called allostatic load, the body is unable to return biological levels to their norm.

Because stress is part of the body's reaction to any threat (known as the fight or flight response) the inflammatory response is primed ready for action. While you may consciously know that your life is not at risk most of the time that you are stressed, your brain doesn't necessarily know that.

The response in the brain is similar to how it would be in a life or death situation. A regular underlying level of stress means that your nervous system is constantly activated, and it is this that can cause chronic inflammation. The additional hormones and other substances remain high for too long and the likelihood of damage to cellular function is increased.

> Declining oestrogen levels during menopause can lead to an increase in inflammation.

Why does the gut flare up?

There is an extensive list of causes for inflammation of the gut, with chronic inflammation being caused by multiple diseases. The gut is teeming with bacteria and is exposed to many threats from the outside environment.

Inflammatory bowel disease (IBD) usually develops when you reach your teenage years or twenties, and the two main types are Crohn's disease and ulcerative colitis. The former is the inflammation of any part of the digestive tract, but most commonly this takes place in the

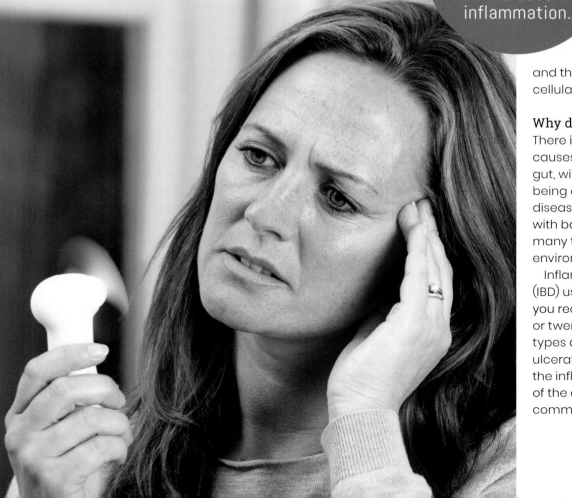

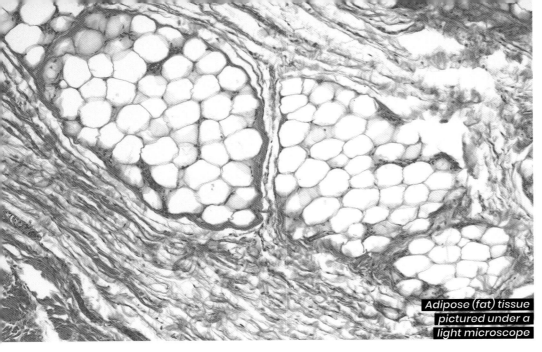

Adipose (fat) tissue pictured under a light microscope

> **Most women witness firsthand how a change in the levels of oestrogen impacts the body**

small intestine and the start of the large intestine.

Scientists are working to find out the exact cause of this unpredictable and painful disease, but in some instances it is genetic. An imbalance in types of gut bacteria can also be the instigator of gut inflammation. The inflammation experienced in Crohn's disease can extend deeper into tissue surrounding the gut, but this isn't the case in inflammation caused by ulcerative colitis.

Ulcerative colitis is the inflammation contained in the lining of the rectum and colon. This condition may be caused as a result of failed immune system responses. When pathogens are detected in this part of the body, the cells that are sent to attack them can also attack the healthy cells lining the gut. If this happens, an additional inflammatory response is activated and the symptoms of abdominal cramping, bleeding and pain begin.

The genetics of inflammation

In 2016, 50 research centres around the world collectively discovered hundreds of genes that are responsible for inflammatory diseases. The large-scale, worldwide study focused on the following inflammatory diseases: ankylosing spondylitis, Crohn's Disease, ulcerative colitis, psoriasis and primary sclerosing cholangitis.

As conditions that impact around 3% of the global population, the purpose of the study was to work out how these diseases could be controlled. Is there a collective environmental cause that is affecting so many people, or are these outcomes largely predetermined in a person's genetic makeup?

The research analysed the circumstances of 86,000 participants from 26 different countries. As a result, 244 genetic variants were found to be determining factors of these inflammatory diseases.

Hormone levels: testosterone and oestrogen

The levels of the two main sex hormones, testosterone (male) and oestrogen (female) can influence the likelihood of inflammation in the body. This is due to one of the many roles of testosterone. The hormone plays an essential role in preventing the accumulation of too much fatty tissue.

Studies have found a link between low testosterone levels and the emergence of chronic inflammatory disease. Obesity is a significant contributor to some inflammatory diseases, and testosterone level is closely related to body fat mass. For those whose testosterone levels are low and who are struggling with weight-related health issues, testosterone therapy is sometimes suggested. This has been shown to help people shed body fat and lead healthier lives. Testosterone replacement demonstrates that it can reduce inflammation in the process.

Low levels of oestrogen has a similar outcome in the body when it comes to inflammation. Most women witness firsthand how a change in the levels of oestrogen impacts the body. After menopause, which signals the end of the menstrual cycle, women have a higher white blood cell count than beforehand. Scientists think this is primarily due to an underlying increase in inflammation.

Before menopause, high levels of oestrogen in the female body help to maintain the reproductive system. After the childbearing years are over, the need for this level of oestrogen isn't necessary – at least not for the same purposes. As the anti-inflammatory hormone declines, women become slightly more susceptible to inflammation in the joints, cardiovascular, cognitive and gut inflammation.

The impact of exercise

Physical activity is associated with good health. And in the case of inflammation, there is little exception. Moderate exercise strengthens the circulation of blood around the body, making the inflammatory response more efficient when it is needed. Knowing your limit when it comes to exercise is essential, especially if your purpose is to reduce inflammation. Too much high-intensity exercise can have the opposite effect, by causing damage to muscle and connective tissue. This causes inflammation of the damaged area, reversing any benefits that were gained by keeping fit.

Of all the causes of inflammation, some are in your control to manage, while others are unpreventable. Exercising moderately, adding anti-inflammatory foods to your meals, and finding time to destress are some of the easy ways to reduce general inflammation on a daily basis.

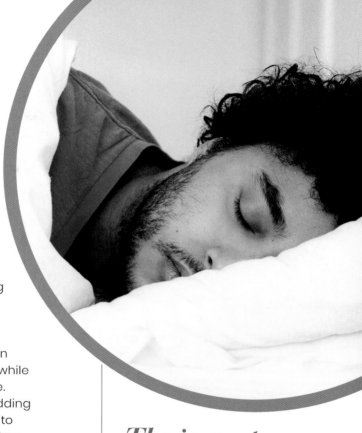

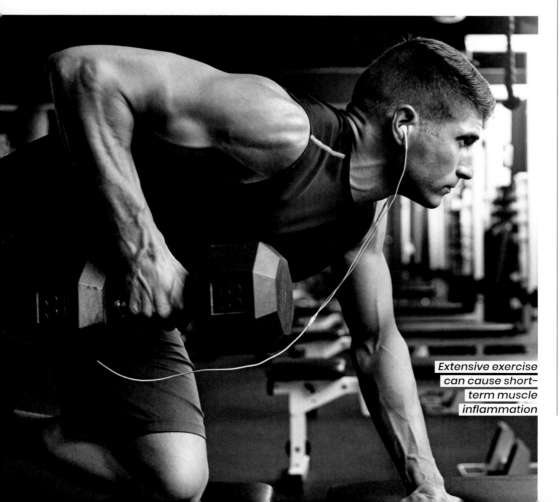

Extensive exercise can cause short-term muscle inflammation

The importance of a good night's sleep

Whenever you become unwell, you may have noticed the constant urge to sleep. During sleep, your body's physical demands are reduced and it can use all its energy to attack infection at a cellular level. If you don't get enough rest, sleep deprivation produces a higher number of inflammation molecules into the blood.

People who attain less sleep each night are more prone to developing diabetes, high blood pressure, cardiovascular disease and many chronic inflammatory conditions. When you wake up after a deep sleep, your mind is clearer, literally. Cerebrospinal fluid passes through your brain during some of the deepest stages of sleep like a filter, removing many inflammatory proteins.

DIAGNOSING
inflammation

These are some of the signs that your body is in inflammatory attack mode

The four main indicators of inflammation – pain, swelling, heat and redness – portray a very limited picture of what inflammation looks like. In reality, there are many varying realities for each of these four symptoms, depending on the level of inflammation and where it is occurring in the body.

Some forms of inflammation are easy to self-diagnose when you are aware of the symptoms. Others, such as inflammation of certain internal organs and diseases triggered by specific substances in the blood, need to be analysed by a doctor for accurate diagnostics. Knowing the general feelings that may arise during and after episodes of inflammation means that you can look out for some of the

There are about 36,000 MRI machines around the world.

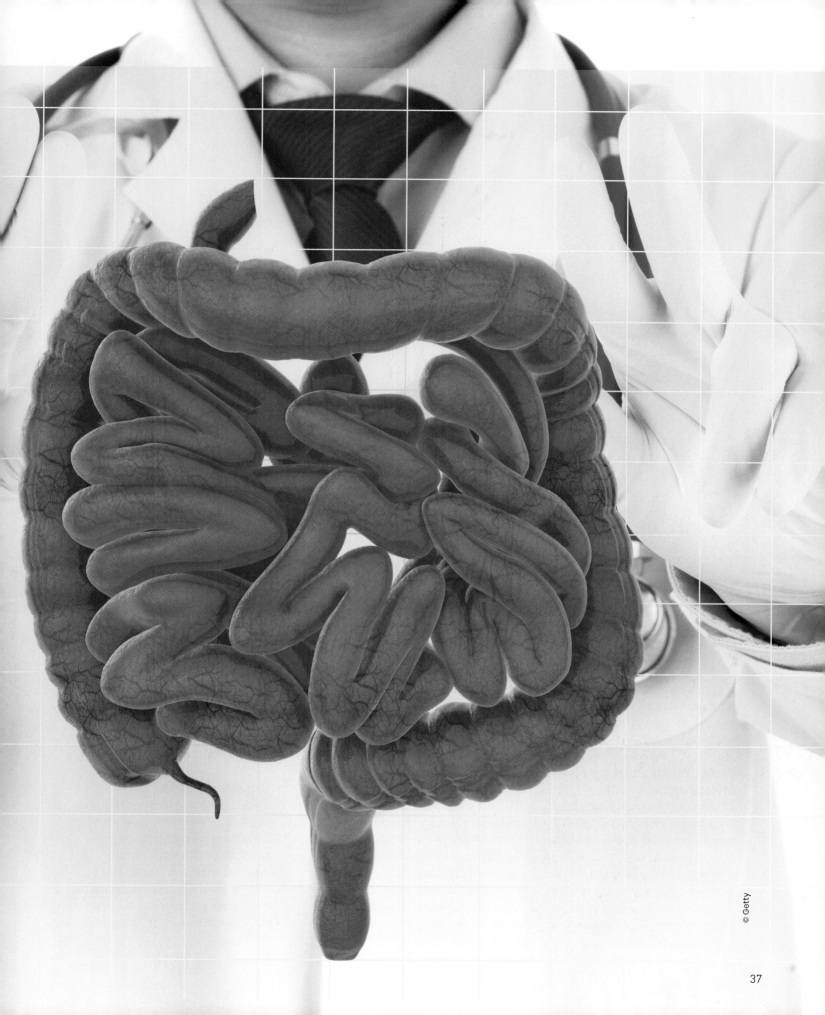

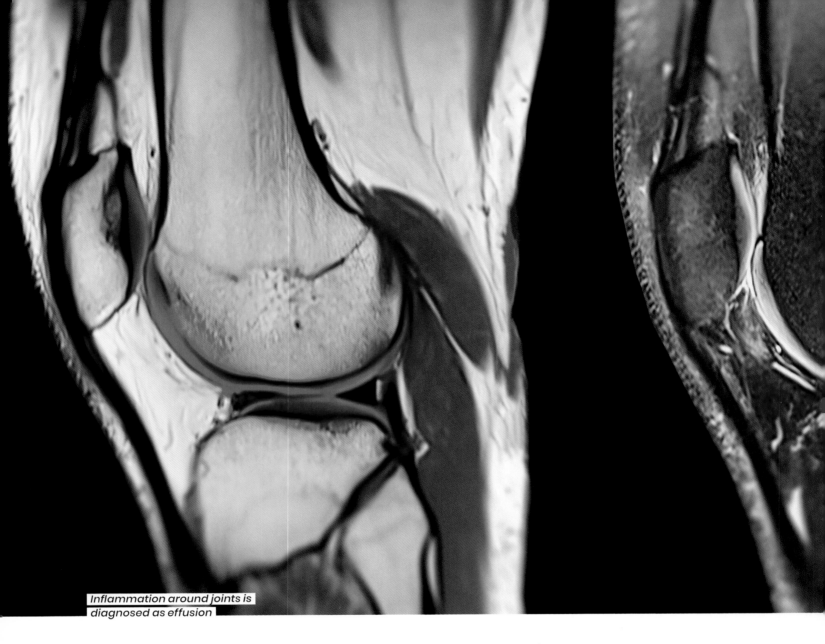

Inflammation around joints is diagnosed as effusion

telltale signs of inflammation and seek professional help to find out the precise root cause of unusual symptoms. This is how different forms of inflammation are diagnosed.

Detecting inflammation after physical trauma

When you fall or get hit by an object, any swelling that is produced will emerge after the pain. Pain is almost always the first sign of inflammation to be diagnosed, and it exists for that reason. Humans have evolved to feel pain so that we become aware of a problem in the body and can try to avoid any further damage.

If inflammation occurs after an event of physical trauma, the swelling can either be diagnosed as edema or effusion. Edema is the term used to describe any swelling that is located outside of a joint. This is the common inflammatory response, caused by the leakage of fluid and white blood cells from blood vessels into the tissue.

Alternatively, injury caused by a blunt impact to joints is likely to be effusion. Effusion is the inflammation that arises in or around a joint. If your pain and swelling is located in areas such as the knee or ankle, then injury to bones, tendons, ligaments or cartilage in the joint area could be causing the swelling.

Signs on the skin

If you develop a rash on the surface of the body, this could be a symptom of a huge number of skin inflammatory causes. To narrow down the trigger for the outbreak, a doctor might ask you when the rash appeared and what you were

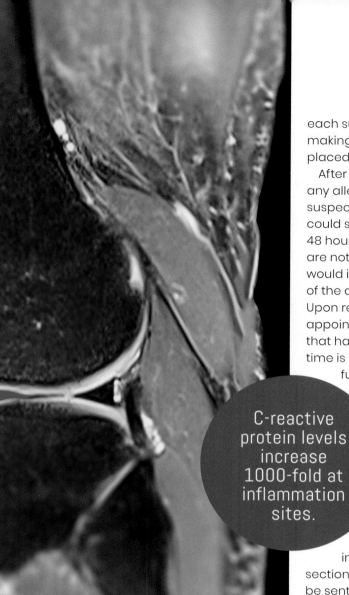

each substance into the back, making a note of which was placed where.

After exposing your body to any allergens that the doctor suspects to be the cause, they could send you home for up to 48 hours. During this time you are not allowed to wash, as that would interfere with the results of the diagnostic experiment. Upon returning to the follow-up appointment, any inflammation that has emerged during this time is noted as an allergen to be further explored.

If the inflammatory reaction was more severe, and the doctor doesn't want to risk exposing the skin to this danger again in a skin test, a biopsy may be used instead. This involves removing a small section of the skin so that it can be sent to a laboratory for testing and close examination under a microscope.

C-reactive protein levels increase 1000-fold at inflammation sites.

doing beforehand. What you were eating, any activities you were participating in, and the environment you were in when the inflammation occurred are all relevant as potential causes.

To test for potential allergies that might have caused skin inflammation, blood can be taken and tested, or your doctor might suggest a skin test. Often, the test is carried out on the skin of the back, as the large surface area means that multiple allergens can be tested. In a grid-shaped pattern, the doctor will inject a small amount of

What does blood vessel inflammation feel like?

The first signs that you might be suffering from vasculitis – the name given to any inflammation of the blood vessels – are headaches, tiredness, fevers, weight loss, aches and pains. Because all these symptoms are very general, and relate to so many health issues, a true diagnosis has to come from a medical professional.

Inflammation of the blood vessels in the eyes and ears can cause dizziness, as well as ringing in the ears or sight

5 common conditions misdiagnosed as bowel inflammation

Sarcoidosis
This condition usually causes swollen tissue to clump together in the lungs and skin. However, in less than 1% of cases, sarcoidosis symptoms are felt in the abdomen.

Behcet's disease
This inflammation of blood vessels and tissues usually causes ulcers in the mouth and genitals. Sometimes it can be found in the intestines, mimicking Crohn's disease.

Diverticulitis
Diverticulitis has similar symptoms to ulcerative colitis. It produces inflamed pouches along the intestinal lining instead of the ulcers seen in ulcerative colitis.

Coccidioides
This is a fungal infection that most often targets the lungs, causing inflammation. As it isn't associated with the intestines, it can be misdiagnosed as an IBD when it infects them.

Campylobacter
This bacterium makes its way to the intestines when ingested with food. It produces abdominal pain, fever and diarrhoea, which are similar symptoms to those of IBDs.

© Getty

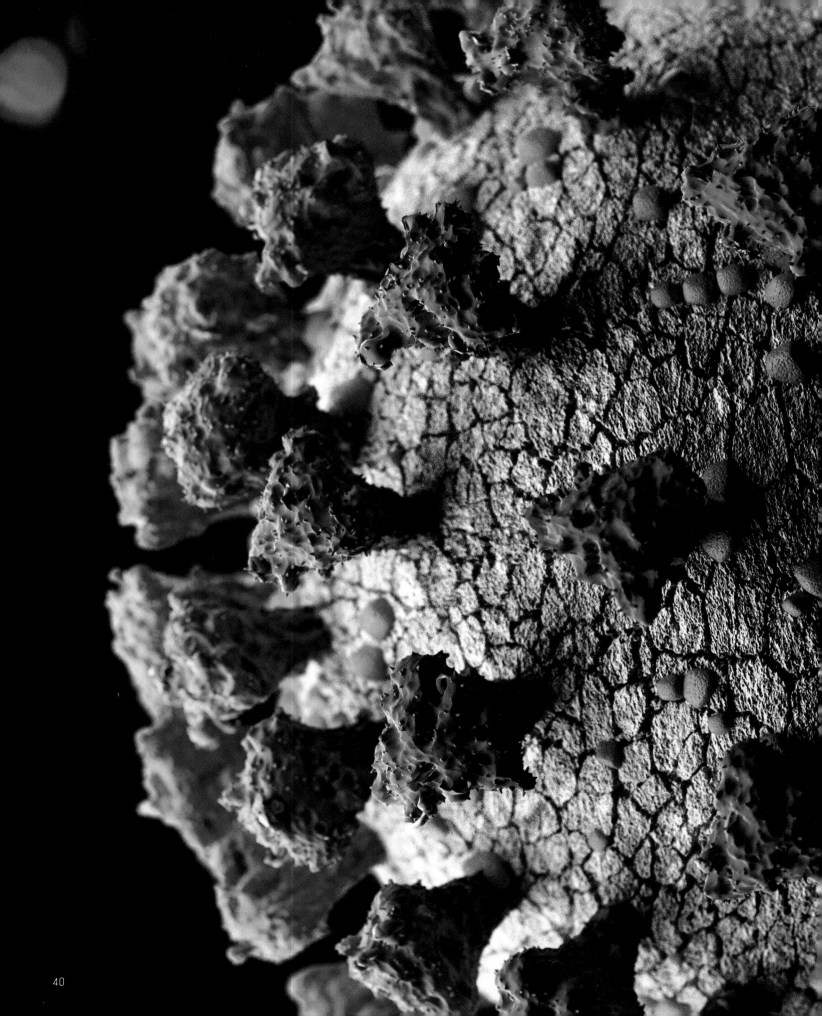

> ## The first signs of heart inflammation can be picked up by doctors after listening to your chest with a stethoscope

loss and itchy, burning eyes. If the blood vessels in your hands or feet are inflamed, the skin on the palms of the hands or soles of the feet can become swollen and hardened.

Vasculitis is detected more thoroughly through either blood tests, imaging tests, biopsies or angiographies. Imaging tests are useful for displaying a clear picture of individual blood vessels and determining which are inflamed, as well as any impacted organs. Computerised tomography (CT), magnetic resonance imaging (MRI), X-rays, ultrasound and positron emission tomography (PET) are all viable imaging methods for this diagnosis.

Angiographies are similar to X-rays, but are used when a clear view of blood vessels is required. This can't be obtained from a standard X-ray. Before the scan, a special dye is inserted into the bloodstream. This produces definite outlines of the blood vessels in the final images.

If the inflammation in the blood vessels has progressed enough to cause the vessel walls to balloon outwards, you might be recommended for surgery. This is to reduce the chance of the inflamed blood vessels rupturing.

Do you have a healthy heart?

Any evidence of compromised heart function is taken incredibly seriously by medical professionals. If inflammation is occurring in the heart, you might experience chest pain, swelling in the lower parts of the body as circulation is compromised, light-headedness or shortness of breath.

The first signs of heart inflammation can be picked up by doctors after listening to your chest with a stethoscope. Using this device, they can hear the movement of blood flowing through the heart. One indication of inflammation in or around the organ is that the beating sound is more scratchy than would be expected in a healthy heart.

One of the most detailed machine images used to reveal the inflammatory situation within the heart is a cardiac MRI machine. Using radio waves and magnetic fields, the size, structural elements and changes in shape due to inflammation will be displayed. In particular, this method reveals inflamed heart muscle.

Diagnosing IBDs

Crohn's disease and ulcerative colitis, the two main inflammatory bowel diseases (IBDs), are almost impossible to diagnose yourself, due to them presenting almost identical symptoms. You

A NEW DIAGNOSIS

Along with the emergence of COVID-19 in late 2019, some children began to display serious symptoms of inflammation after contracting the coronavirus. For the majority of children who caught the virus, only mild cold-like symptoms were experienced. But cases of children reacting much more seriously to the virus soon began to emerge. In 2020, this new condition was given a name: multisystem inflammatory syndrome (MIS-C).

MIS-C is a serious syndrome that can cause the heart, lungs, blood vessels, brain, skin, eyes, digestive system or kidneys to suffer from significant inflammation. The symptoms of the syndrome vary due to the many areas of the body that can be targeted. Because it is a newly developed condition, brought about by COVID-19, scientists' knowledge of it is limited. That is why it is currently classed as an inflammatory syndrome, rather than an inflammatory disease. MIS-C remains rare, and MIS-A (a similar syndrome that occurs in adults) is even rarer, emerging weeks after being infected with the COVID-19 virus.

can, however, look for general signs of bowel inflammation, and closer inspection reveals which IBD is the cause. Abdominal pain, bloating and any changes in bowel habits or the stool itself are indications of an inflammatory response in the digestive tract.

During the differentiation process between Crohn's disease and ulcerative colitis, a medical professional will likely need to collect stool and blood samples from you. Most commonly, a colonoscopy is performed to see what is happening inside the intestines. The flexible camera, which is inserted into the intestines, can spot any bleeding, polyps – which are small growths protruding from the inner lining of the intestines – and signs of cancer. By observing where the inflammation is taking place,

> ## 66
> ## The first signs of heart inflammation can be picked up by doctors after listening to your chest with a stethoscope

doctors can diagnose either ulcerative colitis (in the colon) or Crohn's disease (if inflammation is in another part of the digestive tract).

Detecting other causes of digestive inflammation
Of course, not all causes of digestive inflammation are chronic diseases. Inflammation can be caused by temporary situations, such as the presence of gallstones or pathogens. To get a closer look at the entire digestive tract, and see where inflammation is occurring, you might be asked to record a short film of your insides, in the form of a capsule endoscopy.

A capsule endoscopy involves swallowing a camera the size of a large pill. Inside this is at least one camera, along with a light and transmitter. Unlike the fate of your food, the sealed capsule can't be broken down by the enzymes and other activity during digestion. Instead, the camera captures two images every second, for the several hours that it takes to pass through the body, and the series of images are transmitted and stored to a computer for analysis. In most cases, the camera is

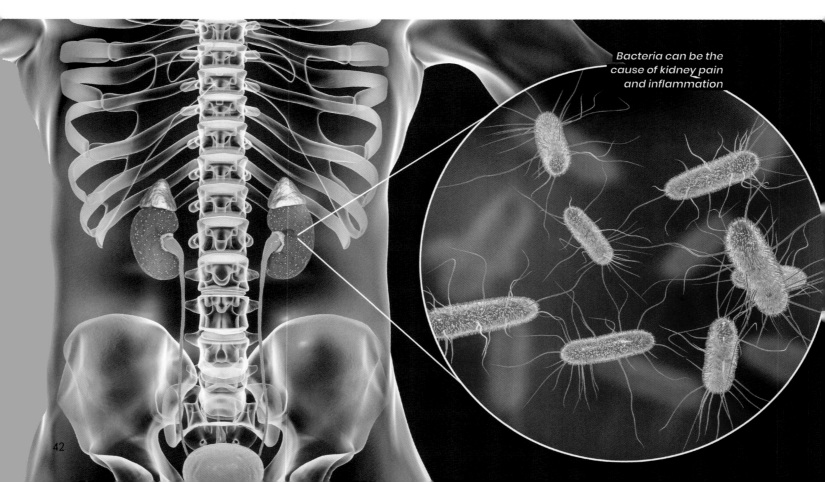

Bacteria can be the cause of kidney pain and inflammation

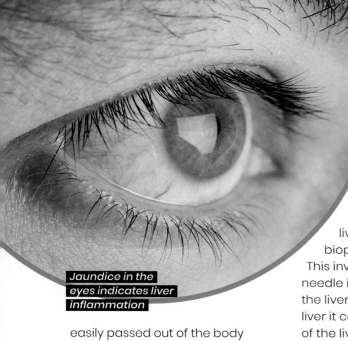

Jaundice in the eyes indicates liver inflammation

easily passed out of the body naturally within 24 hours.

What does an enlarged liver look like?

When your liver becomes inflamed, it can present some general symptoms, as well as more specific signs, that your organ has become enlarged. One of the more obvious signs is jaundice. This condition causes your skin, and the white parts of your eyes, to turn yellow. Other more general signs of an enlarged liver are feeling full soon into a meal, nausea, abdominal pain and fatigue.

To diagnose an inflamed liver, the first step that a healthcare professional will take is to physically feel the abdomen. Depending on how inflamed the organ is, a doctor might be able to notice swelling in the area of the liver, externally. In most cases, additional steps will need to be taken, though.

Blood tests are used to measure the activity levels of liver enzymes. In an inflamed liver, these enzymes are sure to increase in the blood, sometimes noticeably when pictured next to other organs. CT and MRI scans are also used, as they can show the outline of the organ and how its size compares with other anatomical features.

If medical professions want to take a look at the liver cells close up, a liver biopsy can be performed. This involves inserting a long needle into the skin until it hits the liver. As the needle enters the liver it cores out a minute section of the liver and removes it from the body. The cells are sent to the laboratory for testing, and can provide clear answers about the cause of inflammation.

Kidneys: pain in the pelvis

Depending on the cause of kidney inflammation, the first signs can vary. However, there are key symptoms to look out for that cover the majority of cases. First, pain in the pelvic area and abdomen is likely to develop. In some cases, this pain is limited to the sides of the abdomen, near where these organs are located.

Due to the kidneys' role of filtering out toxic

This small endoscope camera records your insides when swallowed

substances to pass in the urine, the process of urinating itself can aid the diagnosis. Urinating should be a pain-free experience, but when the kidneys are inflamed, urinating might result in a burning sensation or pain being felt.

Inflammation in these organs can also increase how frequently you need to urinate, and might result in blood or pus in the urine, or cloudy urine. When kidneys fail to effectively remove excess fluid from the body, indications of inflammation can arise elsewhere in the form of swelling. The accumulation of fluid gathers in the face, legs and feet most commonly.

To diagnose kidney inflammation, doctors look for substance concentrations in the blood and urine. If blood, bacteria or white blood cells are found in the urine, or high concentrations of toxins that should have been removed by the kidneys are discovered circulating in the blood, you will receive a diagnosis of kidney inflammation.

Breathing with lung inflammation

Any form of inflammation in the lungs impacts your ability to exchange gases through the tissue and breathe optimally. The most obvious signs of this are difficulty

> There have been more than 7,000 reported cases of MIS-C in the United States.

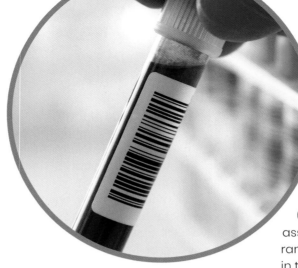

HOW CAN DOCTORS TEST YOUR BLOOD?

Blood tests are one of the most common procedures used to diagnose inflammation. Because inflammation occurs as a response in the blood, evidence is most often retrieved there. A higher concentration of inflammatory proteins are found in the blood following inflammation. As damaged cells launch an inflammatory response, extra protein is released at the site. Erythrocyte sedimentation rate (ESR), C-reactive protein (CRP) and plasma viscosity (PV) blood tests are the three main blood tests used. ESR tests measure the rate of red blood cell separation from the plasma. The extracted blood is placed into an upright tube. Separated blood cells will then be seen falling to the bottom of the tube and the volume of plasma collected after a given time is recorded. High levels of inflammatory proteins cause the red blood cells to stick together and separate at a quicker rate. CRP is a specific protein that is released during inflammation. Higher concentrations of this protein show high levels of inflammation. If high levels of protein are circulating the body, then the extracted blood will show a highly viscous plasma. Each of these types of blood tests are nonspecific, so won't show where the inflammation is taking place. However, they are reliable for proving that inflammation is present.

breathing, sounds of wheezing when inhaling or chest pain and tightness.

Because there are so many causes for lung inflammation, ranging in severity, the diagnostic process is a series of tests used to narrow down the specific cause and locate the exact location of inflammation. First, though, a doctor needs to check if the threat is an emergency. For immediate threats, treatment is needed, while chronic diseases are diagnosed with methods for day-to-day management.

In the first diagnostic tests, a doctor will watch you breathe. If breathing is short and sharp, or the neck muscles are needed to assist in the intake of air, these are signs that inflammation of the lungs is preventing natural breathing. A non-invasive sensor may be placed onto the tip of your finger to measure how much oxygen is passing through the blood vessels. This is called a pulse oximeter and, when low levels of oxygen are detected, lung function is likely to be compromised. Eventually, inflammation is confirmed after

High blood-sugar levels can be diagnosed with home-testing finger-prick kits.

a CT scan of the chest reveals the abnormality.

Which part of the brain is inflamed?

Brain inflammation (encephalitis) causes an assortment of symptoms, ranging from pain and stiffness in the head and neck area to confusion, irritability and loss of consciousness. Being a vital and delicate organ, which can significantly alter a person's mental capabilities if injury persists, scans are usually recommended soon after symptoms arise.

The two main brain scans are MRI and CT scans, which give doctors clear images – taken from all angles – of any tumours or swelling. CT scans are quicker than MRI scans, but the finer details of the brain's soft tissue are less evident. So, when the prevalence of inflammation needs to be detected on a time scale, CTs are best for diagnosis. But, when finer details are required, MRI scans are more likely to be used.

Inflammation of a singular area of the brain can be a sign of injury or tumours, while general enlargement of brain tissue may be due to infection. Electroencephalograms (EEGs) are used to monitor any suspicious behaviour in brain activity. Electrodes are stuck to a patient's scalp and the electrical

> ## Brain inflammation causes symptoms ranging from pain and stiffness in the head and neck area to confusion and irritability

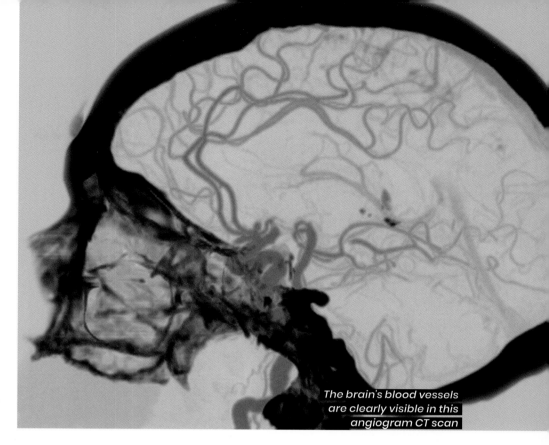

The brain's blood vessels are clearly visible in this angiogram CT scan

activity is presented on a digital screen. Unusual findings indicate encephalitis.

Diagnosis of brain infections can be confirmed by attaining tissue from the body. This diagnosis doesn't have to involve touching the delicate tissues of the brain. Instead, fluid that surrounds the spine can be extracted. This is called cerebrospinal fluid (CSF) and is the same as that found in the brain. Plus, extracting fluid from this area is much safer than going near the brain. Brain biopsies can be performed as a last resort, if symptoms begin to worsen and treatment isn't proving effective.

Called a spinal tap, removing cerebrospinal fluid is as easy as inserting a needle into the lower back. Any differences in this fluid, compared to what is expected in a healthy individual, can be used to diagnose inflammatory brain diseases.

Why is early diagnosis essential?

While acute inflammation can be left alone, and inflamed areas heal by themselves after cellular response, chronic inflammation should be diagnosed as early as possible. The longer that chronic inflammation is left untreated, the higher the chance of complications emerging. Some inflammatory conditions, such as arthritis, can be completely reversed if treated in the earliest stages.

The detriment caused by chronic inflammation to surrounding tissues increases as time goes on. This can cause internal scarring, tissue death and DNA damage. Knowing the signs of inflammation greatly reduces your chances of developing other illnesses as a result. As inflammation increases your risk of heart disease, cancer and other serious illnesses, many patients are completely oblivious to inflammation until another illness is diagnosed.

One of the main benefits of diagnosis, at any stage, is that treatment can be arranged to reduce pain. The bottom line is that if you are experiencing any of the signs of inflammation, you should seek medical advice as soon as possible. This will either rule out serious inflammation or provide solutions to enhance your life in the present and future.

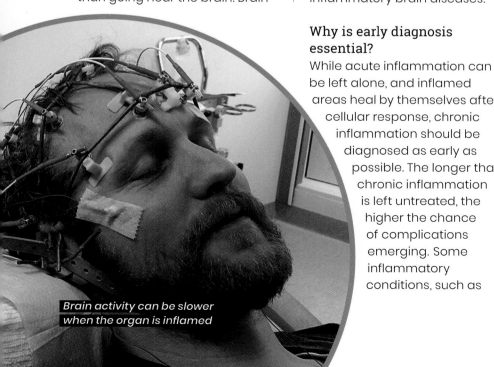

Brain activity can be slower when the organ is inflamed

LIFESTYLE

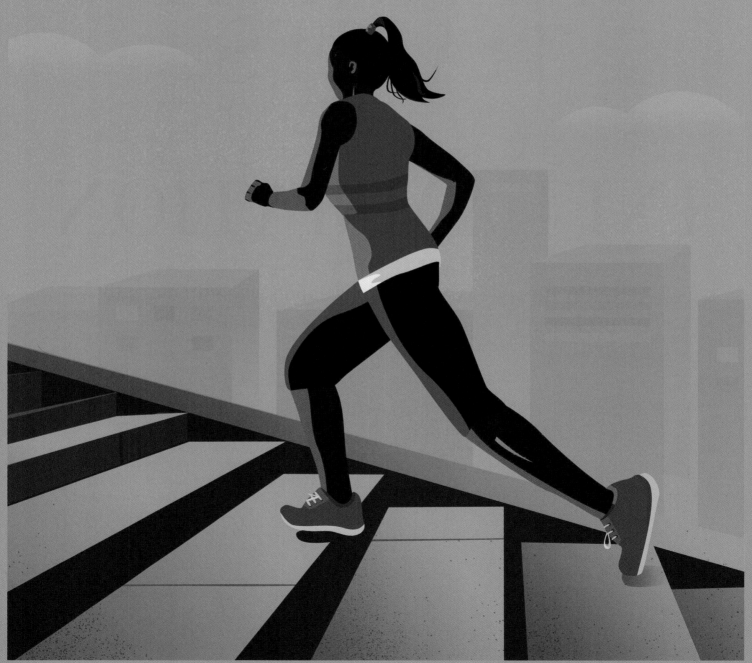

Hello HEALTHY HABITS, GOODBYE INFLAMMATION

A healthy lifestyle is a powerful weapon when it comes to preventing, controlling and reducing inflammation

While a stressful, sedentary lifestyle and highly processed diet can cause or contribute to unhealthy inflammation, reversing these trends addresses the problem. Good nutrition, sleep, exercise and reducing stress levels are the fab four when it comes to fighting back, as we'll look at in more depth in the features to come.

You are what you eat

One of the first priorities is to achieve, or maintain, a healthy weight through a balanced diet. There are proven links between weight gain and increased inflammation, with obesity found to cause low-grade chronic inflammation.

Some foods and ways of eating (like the Mediterranean diet) are known for having specific anti-inflammatory qualities, while others can actively increase it and are best avoided or limited. "Eating a rainbow of food from green leafy vegetables to brightly coloured fresh fruit provides the body with vital antioxidants and phyto-nutrients that target inflammation," says nutritionist and author Barbara Cox-Lovesy (www.barbaracox.me).

"Plan your meals to include a wide variety of colourful foods that vary daily and make the most of the anti-inflammatory properties of spices like turmeric, pepper, ginger and garlic."

A diet based on fruits, vegetables, nuts, whole grains, fish and healthy oils is seen as one of the best anti-inflammatory eating plans, according to experts at the Harvard School of Public Health.

Exercise your options

Regular exercise provides multiple benefits in warding off inflammation. Not only does it play a part in keeping us at a healthy weight, but it also helps reduce stress and increases the likelihood of a good night's sleep. In addition to aerobic exercise and weight or resistance training, consider taking up yoga. A review of numerous research studies that covered a range of different yoga styles, found that all were effective in reducing inflammation across a range of chronic conditions.

"High stress levels play a big part in inflammation and yoga is a practice known to reduce these," adds yoga teacher and Thai yoga massage therapist Penelope Zikic, who is based at triyoga, Chelsea and Camden in the UK (www.triyoga.co.uk). "The focus on breath, essential in all yoga practices, helps to calm and balance the body's parasympathetic and sympathetic nervous system, which helps regulate stress levels and encourages relaxation."

If you are trying to give up smoking, avoid turning to e-cigarettes.

A 2018 study found the vapour boosts inflammation

Chill out

While stress is normal, being in perpetual fight or flight mode isn't what our bodies were designed for. Long-term exposure to the stress hormones cortisol and adrenaline suppresses our immune system. That then results in an inflammatory response.

Other ways of managing stress include guided imagery, massage, time spent outdoors and meditation. A review of a range of trials involving more than 800 participants carried out at Coventry University's Brain, Belief and Behaviour lab, found that genes linked to inflammation became less active in those involved in mind-body practices. These include yoga, tai chi and meditation. Another 2016 study found regular meditators had lower levels of cortisol and reduced inflammatory responses.

Sleep soundly

Modern life throws us many distractions when it comes to getting a good night's sleep. But being sleep-deprived is proven to play a significant part in the inflammatory process. One theory for this is that blood pressure drops during sleep, and restricting the amount of shut-eye that we get means that it doesn't decline as it should. In response, this then triggers cells in blood vessel walls that activate inflammation.

Short on time?

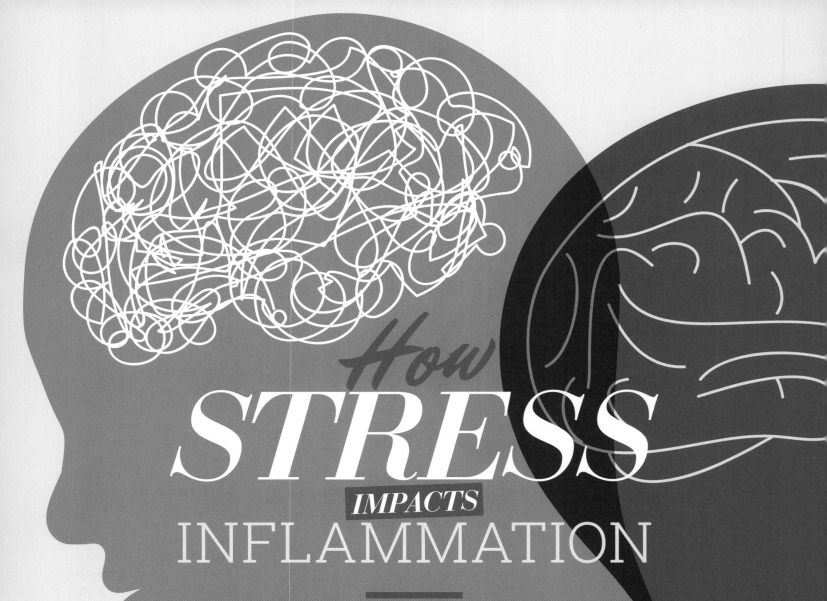

How STRESS IMPACTS INFLAMMATION

Chronic stress can lead to chronic inflammation. We look at why this happens and how to handle it

We all feel stressed at times. It's a normal reaction when things in our life are trying or difficult. A small amount of stress can even be beneficial, pushing us out of our comfort zone or helping us to excel at work. Stress can help us manage every day, juggling work, home and family life.

In this way, stress is a lot like inflammation. A small amount of it from time to time is a normal, healthy and natural reaction in the body to external influences. But, just like inflammation, too much stress over a long period of time can cause significant problems. Too much stress can affect everything from our mood and our bodies, to the way we interact with people around us, like our family or colleagues. Lots of stress over a long period of time can push us towards

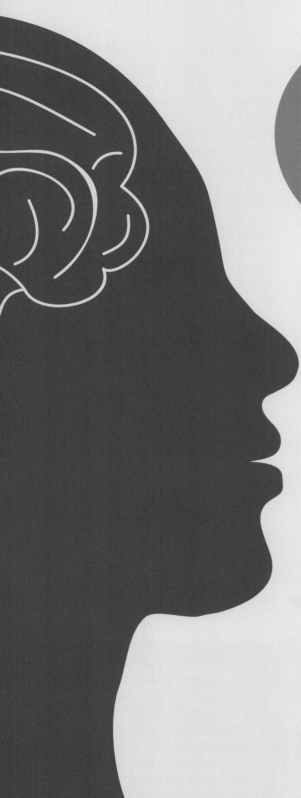

Keep a notebook in your bag and write down anything that's worrying you when it pops up, so you don't have to think about it there and then.

Learning to control our stress levels is an important way to combat stress-related inflammation

'burnout', which is when we're physically, emotionally and mentally exhausted, and no longer feel like we can cope.

Stress can often be normalised, and considered a part of everyday life. However, chronic long-term stress is a real problem that needs to be dealt with. Stress can bring with it some physical symptoms, such as a faster heartbeat, headaches, sore muscles and joints, tiredness and digestive issues. It also hugely impacts on your mental state, causing you to lose focus, struggle to concentrate, have memory problems, feel low or anxious, and affect your self-esteem. We are all different, so you might experience some of these symptoms (or different ones), but not others. Chronic stress can impact a great deal on day-to-day life, and this is when you need to get some help in managing your stress levels before it goes any further.

Stress is also linked to the level of inflammation in our body. Stress is a physical response to feeling threatened. You might have heard of the 'fight or flight' response – your body detects

Signs of stress

Look out for the symptoms so you know when it's time to take action

Struggling to sleep, but feeling tired
Stress can make you feel exhausted and yet often sleep doesn't come easily, especially if you're worrying or having trouble switching off.

Feeling overwhelmed
You might find that you're struggling to control your thoughts and worries, with your brain feeling like it's going into overdrive and racing. This can lead to being overwhelmed.

Eating or drinking more or less
Stress can impact on your food and drink habits, but not always in the same way. Some people find that they eat larger quantities of food, or drink more alcohol when they're under a lot of stress, whereas others lose their appetite.

Being snappy or irritable
When you're stressed and preoccupied with worry, you might find that you're short or irritable with other people. This can especially be true around people you live with or those you are close to.

Avoiding usual activities
You may find that when you're under stress, you withdraw from your normal social life and seeing friends, instead choosing to spend time alone at home.

a threat or challenge, and prepares to combat it. This includes suppressing any body functions it doesn't need in that moment, such as digestion and immunity. The body produces more cortisol, which triggers the release of energy and can raise blood sugar levels. The body also releases adrenaline, increasing your heart rate to get more oxygen in. In short, the body is ready and primed to fight off or run away from the perceived threat. But, of course, there isn't a real threat. So these functions have been called into action when they're not needed.

Usually, once the threat has passed, the body will return to its normal state. In the case of chronic stress, however, these patterns are repeated over and over again. When we're stressed for long periods of time, we're more susceptible to being ill

and catching viruses, as well as feeling generally run down.

Inflammation is also a physical response to a threat. Therefore, the more time you spend feeling stressed, the more inflammation will be created in your body. Unless you take steps

The more time you spend feeling stressed, the more inflammation will be created

to reduce your stress levels, the body doesn't have the chance to return to its normal, calm state. Studies have shown a link between stress and certain inflammatory conditions, including rheumatoid arthritis, heart disease, inflammatory bowel disease and depression.

Too much inflammation in your body can enhance feelings of stress, so you end up stuck in a perpetual stress-inflammation cycle.

It stands to reason, then, that controlling your stress levels is important in helping to reduce inflammation in your body. Activities that are designed to help us relax and unwind, like gentle exercise or yoga, for example, have been shown to help reduce inflammatory markers in the body.

How to reduce stress

There are lots of ways that you can deal with stress in your life. First, you need to see whether it's possible to remove the things that are causing the stress in your life. Try to write down everything you are worrying about to identify the key areas in your life that are making you feel under pressure. Next, think about what you can do to change these things to make them less stressful. It is not possible to remove all stress triggers – that would be unrealistic – but by at least identifying them and acknowledging them, you can see if there are any small changes that you could make to your life to make things easier.

Quite often we can't change the situation that is causing us

Quick stress relief

If you're in the middle of your day and you feel the stress building up, there are some ways that you can quickly regain some control...

1 If you are able to walk away and go outside for a moment, this can help by removing you from your environment and enabling you to breathe in some fresh air.

2 You may also find that it helps to connect to what's around you when you're feeling very overwhelmed. Try to focus on something you can see, something you can hear, something you can smell, and something you can feel. By tuning in to each sense, it might help to bring you out of a stressed state.

the stress, but we can change the way that we respond to it and how we approach it. For example, if you have a big task that is causing you a lot of stress, can you break it down into more manageable chunks and focus on just one small step at a time? Can you delegate parts of the task to other people? Can you challenge the way you think about the task, and try to reframe it in a more positive light? It's certainly not easy, but sometimes we need to take a step back and start again, especially when we're feeling overwhelmed.

If it's no one thing that is making you feel stressed, but a general build-up of pressure, then you need to look at your lifestyle and what you can do to make yourself feel less stressed day to day. One thing that can work is to practice gratitude on a daily basis. At the beginning or end of each day, try to think about or write down three things that you're grateful for. It can be anything, even something as small as the colours in the sky, or a bird in your garden, or drinking a cup of tea in peace. By focusing on the things we have in our lives, it can help to take the focus off those elements that make us feel stressed.

Leading a healthy, balanced lifestyle can also help us to manage our stress levels. It's been shown that being active and engaging in regular exercise can help manage stress levels. It can burn off the nervous energy and jittery feelings that can build up during a period of stress, but it can also give us time and space to step away from stress and put it into perspective. It doesn't matter what kind of exercise – anything that you enjoy will have benefits. If you can exercise outside, even better! Being out in nature can also relieve the feelings of stress. Try to make sure you get outside every day if you can. Exercise helps to reduce both stress and inflammation, so it is important to make time for it.

If you have a lot of stress in your life, you could try something like meditation. Even five minutes a day can help you to feel less stressed – you could increase the time as you get used to it.

If you can't cope with the stress in your life, it might be time to seek additional help from your doctor or support service. There are talking therapies available that help you to learn strategies to cope with stress, but also to help control your thoughts when you feel like they are racing away from you.

When you learn to manage your stress response, you will also be able to control the level of inflammation caused by it.

> if you know a stressful event is coming up, try to plan what you can, so there's less to worry about.

3 Some people find that having a glass of cold water helps – take the time to drink it slowly. This forces your body to slow down a little, which can stop some of the physical symptoms of stress.

4 Changing your breathing pattern can help too, especially if you are feeling panicked. Take a deep breath in and hold for a few seconds before slowly exhaling; repeat a few times until you feel a little calmer.

How *SLEEP* IMPACTS INFLAMMATION

Find out how the quality and duration of your sleep can have an impact on inflammation in your body

We know what it's like. You're busy with family life, work, exercise, cooking, hobbies, socialising... sleep can take a back seat sometimes. In fact, one in three American adults are not getting enough sleep (according to the Center for Disease Control and Prevention), and one in seven British people survive on dangerously low levels of sleep, under five hours a night (says a study by Direct Line Life Insurance called 'Need for Sleep').

But sleep is important in relation to inflammation and, as such, is a key part in reducing your risk of chronic illness. One study* says that "chronic social threats can drive the development of sleep disturbances in humans, which can contribute to the dysregulation of inflammatory and antiviral responses." Sleep deprivation has been shown to increase certain inflammatory molecules in the body, and lack of sleep has been suggested as a contributory factor towards an increased risk in heart disease, high blood pressure and type 2 diabetes.

Our sleep is linked to our circadian rhythm – physical and mental changes that follow a 24-hour cycle. We also know that this regulates our immune system. If we disrupt our natural rhythm on a regular basis, this can prevent normal immune function and hence increase inflammation in the body. And we're not just talking about long-term sleep conditions here; even one night of bad sleep is enough to cause an inflammatory reaction. It's also thought that women have a higher inflammatory response than men due to lack of sleep – though there aren't enough studies done in this area to determine why that might be.

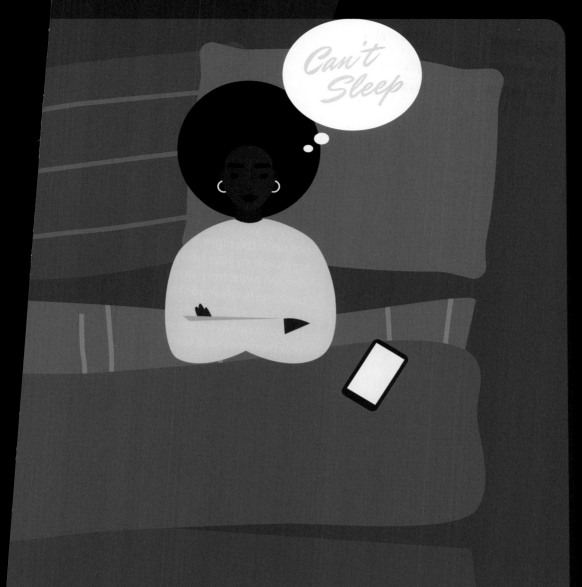

Tips for... *better sleep*

GO TO BED AND WAKE UP AT A REGULAR TIME

LIMIT ALCOHOL AND CAFFEINE AFTER 12PM

Don't eat your meals too late

CREATE A DARK SLEEP ENVIRONMENT

FOLLOW A BEDTIME ROUTINE

GET OUTSIDE DURING THE DAY

Put devices away an hour before bed

your one bad night is isolated, you can usually recover from the increased inflammation with a couple of good nights' sleep. But if you don't sleep enough night after night, then this is when chronic inflammation can occur, along with an increased risk of related illnesses and diseases. You can usually tell when you're starting to suffer from a lack of sleep – you might feel run down or ill, lack concentration, feel unfocused, be unsteady, and have no energy. When we feel like this, we might then be more inclined to eat energy-dense junk foods to perk us up, or skip an exercise session – increasing our levels of inflammation even more.

There are many reasons why you might be finding it hard to sleep. Stress is one of the main causes, and as we look at elsewhere in this book, stress is also a contributory factor towards inflammation. If you're feeling worried or anxious, it's not uncommon to find it hard to switch off and get some sleep. But lack of sleep can in itself be a cause of stress, and so the cycle continues. Sleep not only helps us to control our inflammatory response, but it also helps us to keep our stress under control.

Sleep aids with so many other areas too. For a start, it helps strengthen our immune system and regulates our gut health, both of which can impact on inflammation. If our immune system is being challenged or our gut microbiome is

> ## Most adults need between seven and nine hours of sleep a night

unbalanced, then this will push inflammation in the body even further.

Most adults need between seven and nine hours of sleep a night; you might be further towards one end of the scale than the other. You can usually feel whether you've had enough sleep or too much sleep, but it can be handy to keep a sleep diary for a few months. Log how much sleep you had and how you felt the next day to find the optimum sleep pattern for you.

How to get more sleep

So, now that we know how important sleep is in reducing inflammation, how can you actually improve the duration and quality of your sleep?

First, you need to tune in to your natural sleep/wake cycle, and then work with it. It helps if you can go to bed at roughly the same time each night, and wake up at the same time each day. If you're a shift worker, or have young children, this can be tricky or impossible! It's about doing the best you can – if you have to get up in the night, try to keep the lights low so your body can still discern night from day. Your ideal bedtime is when you're feeling tired enough for sleep – there's no point going to bed early if you then toss and turn trying to get to sleep. You might have to experiment with bedtime to find what works – if you can find the right pattern, you can hopefully wake up naturally in the morning without an alarm clock.

Our body regulates based on light and dark, day and night. Try to make sure that your sleep environment is very dark at night. If you can't block out the external light sources (like streetlights), you might wish to try wearing a sleep mask instead. As you approach your bedtime, start to lower the lights about an hour before, so that it's dim. This will help to prepare

*Sleep and inflammation: partners in sickness and in health, July 2019 **Sleep Disturbance, Sleep Duration, and Inflammation: A Systematic

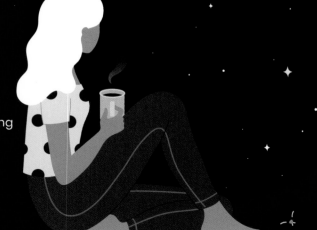

> Going to bed and getting up at the same time every day helps to promote a healthy circadian rhythm.

your mind to switch off and sleep. Then, when it's time to wake up, let the morning light in to signal that the day is starting. It helps if you can get some natural light as soon as possible to tell your body it's time to wake up. It's also good if you can get plenty of time outside during the day. It's hard if you work long hours indoors, but try to get some light from a window or go for a walk in your lunch break. In the winter months it can be difficult to get enough light exposure; you can get lightboxes to help with this if you're really struggling with getting daylight.

Part of controlling your exposure to lights means monitoring and limiting artificial lights too. We are often on our devices late into the evening, but this isn't going to help us wind down. If you can, put your phone away and stop watching television about an hour before bedtime. Try reading (but not on a backlit device) or doing a hobby or craft instead. Keep your phone on silent, or even better in another room, at night so you can't be tempted to look at it.

Exercise and diet can both contribute to good sleep. Aim to do at least 150 minutes of moderate exercise a week, but not too close to your intended bedtime. It's a good idea to add in some relaxing, mindful exercise, like yoga, as well, which can promote relaxation. Eating healthy, balanced foods can also help you to sleep – so an anti-inflammatory diet is perfect for this. Ideally, you don't want to eat too late in the evening, as this can disrupt your sleep while your body works on digesting its last meal. Caffeine can impact your body for much longer than you might think, so try to go caffeine-free after midday or early afternoon.

It takes time to make changes to your sleep routine, but it will pay off in the long run. If you concentrate on your sleep, you will be more likely to feel less stressed, make better food choices, and be more motivated to exercise. Altogether, this will help you commit to your new anti-inflammatory lifestyle.

TOO MUCH SLEEP

While we know that sleep deprivation on a regular basis can play havoc with our bodies and levels of inflammation, did you know that too much sleep can also be problematic? One study in 2016**, found that excessive sleep raised key inflammatory markers, including one specific protein that is linked to heart disease and type 2 diabetes. It can be tempting to catch up on lost sleep at the weekend, but those long lie-ins are doing just as much harm as those shorter nights. It's much better to try to regulate your sleep patterns throughout the week as far as possible, and aim for the right amount of sleep for you to wake up feeling refreshed, focused and energetic. Try to avoid catching up on sleep with naps; it's better to go to bed a bit earlier if you can.

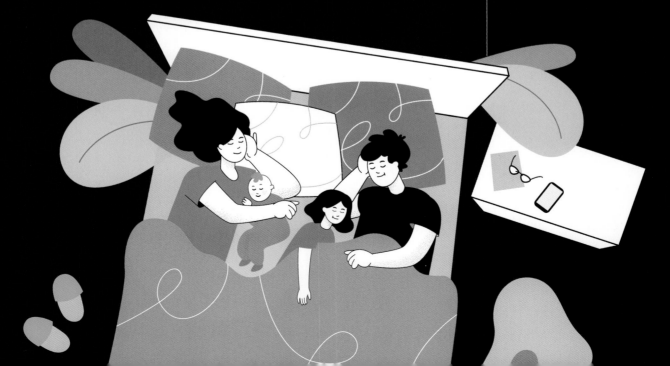

EXERCISE, *weight* & INFLAMMATION

Maintaining a healthy weight and getting enough exercise can help with chronic inflammation

There are many contributory factors when it comes to chronic inflammation in the body. Being overweight, for example, can be a cause of inflammation, as can having a low level of exercise. Sometimes these two factors go hand in hand, but you could be overweight for your body type and get plenty of exercise, or you could have a healthy weight for your body and do no exercise. To maximise the anti-inflammatory benefits, both maintaining a healthy weight and doing enough exercise are important.

Weight and inflammation

Being overweight can put extra stress on the body, and this stress can lead to inflammation. Obesity – a condition in which a person is very overweight, carries a lot of body fat, and has a BMI of over 30 and/or a waist size of over 80 centimetres/31.5 inches (women) or 94 centimetres/37 inches (men) – is linked to an increased risk of heart disease, stroke, type 2 diabetes, certain cancers and 'meta-inflammation'. Meta-inflammation refers to a low-grade chronic inflammation throughout the body, caused by over-nutrition and obesity, and contributes to insulin resistance and metabolic syndrome. You don't need to be suffering from obesity to have enhanced levels of inflammation; even moderate weight gain can impact on your body's inflammatory response.

Losing weight and excess body fat can help to reduce the effects of inflammation. But it's not that simple, or that easy. If you're already in an inflammatory state, it can actually be quite difficult to lose the weight, as the side effects of inflammation, such as insulin resistance, can contribute to weight gain. Many people find that they get stuck in a vicious cycle of being overweight and suffering inflammation. The longer the body has been in a state of inflammation, the harder it can be to reverse the problem.

The first thing that you need is

> Many parks have free outdoor gym equipment – perfect for the summer months!

© Getty

58

patience. Rarely will a quick fix resolve the problem of chronic inflammation. Extreme calorie restriction could cause more stress on the body, and should only be performed under medical supervision. If you are classed as having obesity, then it's worth a chat with your doctor to get professional advice before undertaking a diet.

However, if you're moderately overweight, you can start to move towards a healthy, balanced lifestyle, which will help to reduce inflammation. The way of eating outlined in this book focuses on foods that are nutrient-rich and anti-inflammatory. While the goal of the diet outlined is not primarily to lose weight, many people find that they do drop weight by following the advice given. By cutting out processed, fatty and unhealthy foods, and replacing them with an abundance of fruits, vegetables, lean proteins, healthy fats and wholegrains, you can support your body on its way towards optimum health without going hungry. It does take time to see results, but try to think of it as healing your body from the inside out. As you eat foods that fight inflammation, your body will start to return to a less chronically inflamed state, your blood-sugar levels will stabilise, and your hunger cues will become more balanced.

To lose

5 EXERCISE ACTIVITIES TO REDUCE INFLAMMATION

Walking
Walking is a great, accessible and cheap activity that most of us can do. Make sure you have comfortable shoes and aim for a brisk pace – you should feel a little out of breath and have a slightly elevated heart rate to reap the benefits.

Swimming
This is a great low-impact option if you're new to exercise or you have an injury. It's effective and yet can feel quite relaxing at the same time.

Cycling
The up and down terrain on a typical bike ride challenges your body and is great for your heart! You can adapt it to your current fitness level. Why not combine it with a commute you have to do anyway?

Yoga
Yoga helps with so much, from posture and core strength, to flexibility and relaxation. It has been shown to help with chronic inflammation, by working the body gently and reducing stress.

Home workouts
You don't need a fancy gym or a lot of money to exercise. There are some great workouts online now, many for free, so pick one you like the sound of and give it a go!

weight, you need to eat fewer calories than you expend. That doesn't mean you have to count every calorie, though this works for some people. Most anti-inflammatory food types are naturally lower in calories anyway, and reducing the effects of inflammation can promote weight loss. A food diary can be helpful, whether or not you opt to count calories, as this can help ensure you're getting a good balance of nutrients each day.

Exercise and inflammation

The second part of the puzzle comes down to exercise. Physical exercise has a huge range of benefits, lowering your risk of disease, helping to get to and maintain a healthy weight, and strengthening bones, muscles and the heart. Regular exercise may also support your body's immune system and inflammatory response.

You don't have to do a lot of exercise to reap the benefits either. One study* looked at the benefits of exercise on inflammation. Specifically,

it wanted to see if a single 20-minute session of exercise (in this case walking on a treadmill at moderate intensity) could suppress a certain type of protein, a cytokine called TNF, which has pro-inflammatory properties. TNF is a useful protein that helps induce inflammation when it's needed (such as in the case of injury), but when it comes to chronic inflammation, it can be too abundant. The result of the study showed that just the one single session of moderate exercise did result in an anti-inflammatory response.

This just goes to show that even small changes to your lifestyle could help with inflammation. As with everything, the key is in balance – see our boxout on 'Too much exercise' – and getting the right level of exercise for you. If you're new to exercise, it's best to start slow and build up a little at a time. If you're currently inactive, a good, long-term goal to aim for is the physical activity guidelines set by health bodies around the world. These give a suggested level of exercise that all physically able adults should

aim for, for optimum health and wellbeing.

Most countries have broadly the same guidelines. Aim for at least 150 minutes of moderate exercise or 75 minutes of vigorous exercise (or a combination of both) every week. If you find

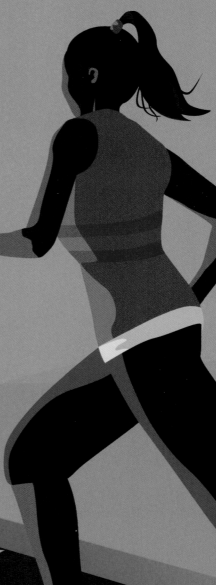

© Getty

> ## Even small changes to your lifestyle could help with inflammation

Try to work exercise into your daily routine – walk instead of driving where possible and take the stairs instead of the lift.

*Inflammation and exercise: Inhibition of monocytic intracellular TNF production by acute exercise via β2-adrenergic activation, March 2017

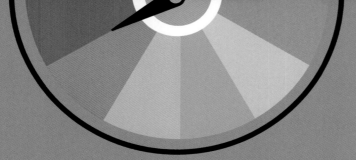

BMI

BMI is a rough gauge to see if you're at a healthy weight for your body type

<16	Severely underweight	25-29.9	Overweight
16-18.4	Underweight	30-34.9	Obesity 1 degree
18.5-24.9	Normal	35-39.9	Obesity 2 degree

something that you enjoy, you're more likely to stick at it. You might prefer to be outside, so try walking at a pace that gets your heart rate up, or running (a Couch to 5K programme is a great place to start). Cycling, team sports, gardening and tennis are all great outdoor pursuits too. If you prefer to be indoors, you could take up swimming, group exercise classes or dance, for example.

Additional to this, adults should also do at least two sessions a week of muscle-strengthening exercise. This could be using assisted or free weights, or bodyweight-based exercise. Often this is the area that gets most overlooked, but it has huge benefits in strengthening your body, promoting weight loss when needed and reducing inflammation. If you're new to weights or bodyweight work, you might wish to join a class or a gym to get some proper instruction. You could even try something like yoga or Pilates,

which are gentle, but do involve a lot of strength work in holding certain positions. These exercises also help with flexibility, which benefits us as we get older.

As well as undertaking exercise, it's also important to move more throughout the day. Many of us have jobs where we have to sit down for long periods of time. Try to get up regularly, just to move the body and stretch, and if you can take a longer walk outside in your lunch break or have an active commute, this all helps too.

If you combine the dietary advice in this book with an increase in your exercise levels, you will find that your body will reduce inflammation, as well as work towards a healthy weight that you can maintain. Not only will this reduce your risk of disease, chronic inflammation and heart conditions, but it can also help you to sleep more deeply and manage stress better – which in turn also helps to reduce inflammation.

TOO MUCH EXERCISE

While a moderate level of exercise is important in helping to reduce inflammation, it is possible to overdo it. If you push yourself at too high an intensity, or exercise too much without adequate rest, you could actually increase the inflammation. This is a normal process; if you push hard, your body needs to repair and heal the muscles. This is why rest days are so key; they give your body the chance to repair everything before your next session. In this case, the inflammation is beneficial and natural. However, the problem comes when you are not giving your body time to repair – if you push too hard, your body is forced to stay in a chronic state of inflammation, which is when the side effects could start to outweigh benefits. Make sure your week is balanced between vigorous and moderate activity, and recovery. Gentle exercise, like walking or yoga, can help your body to heal, so you don't have to do nothing on your rest days.

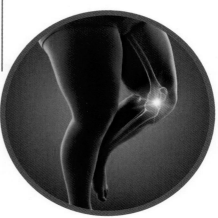

NUTRITION

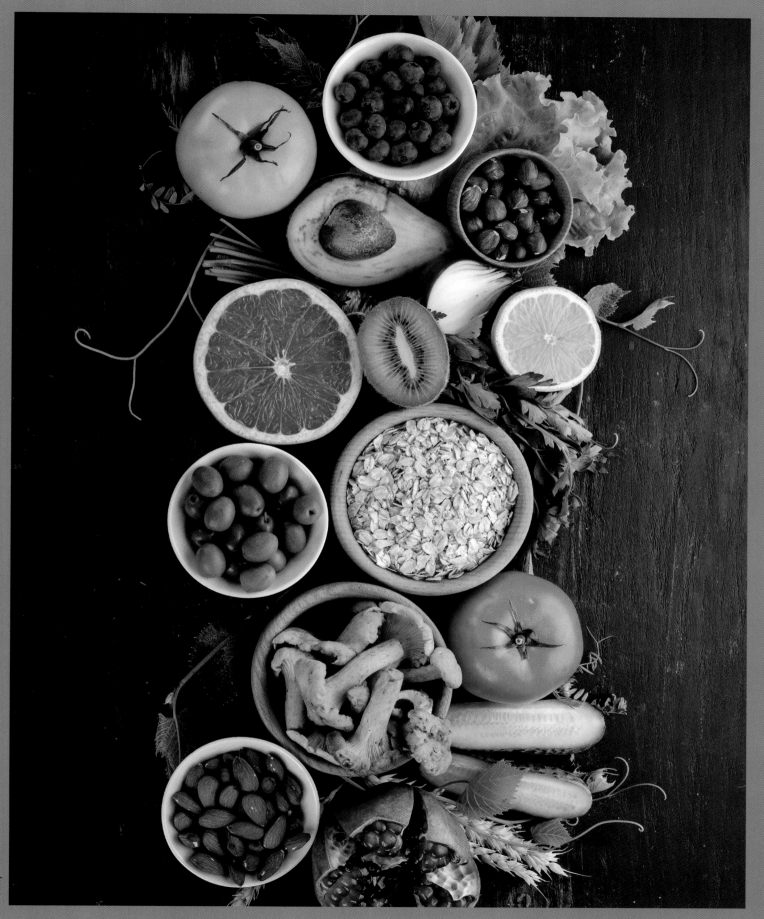

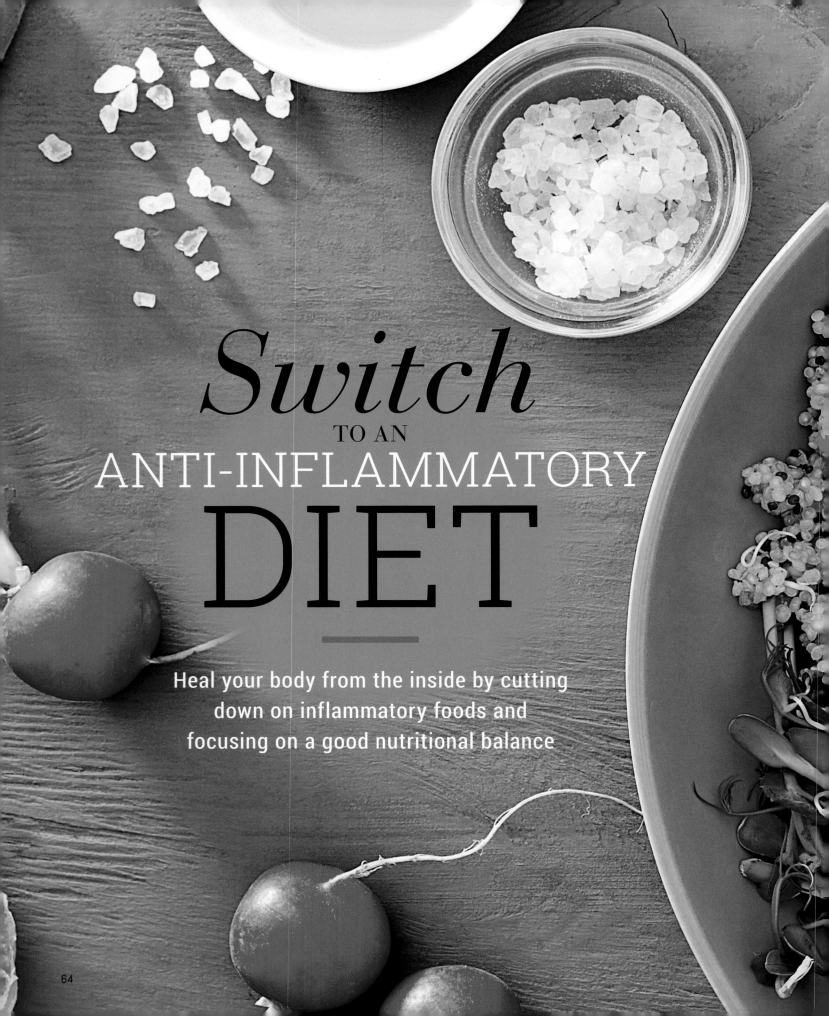

Switch
TO AN
ANTI-INFLAMMATORY
DIET

Heal your body from the inside by cutting
down on inflammatory foods and
focusing on a good nutritional balance

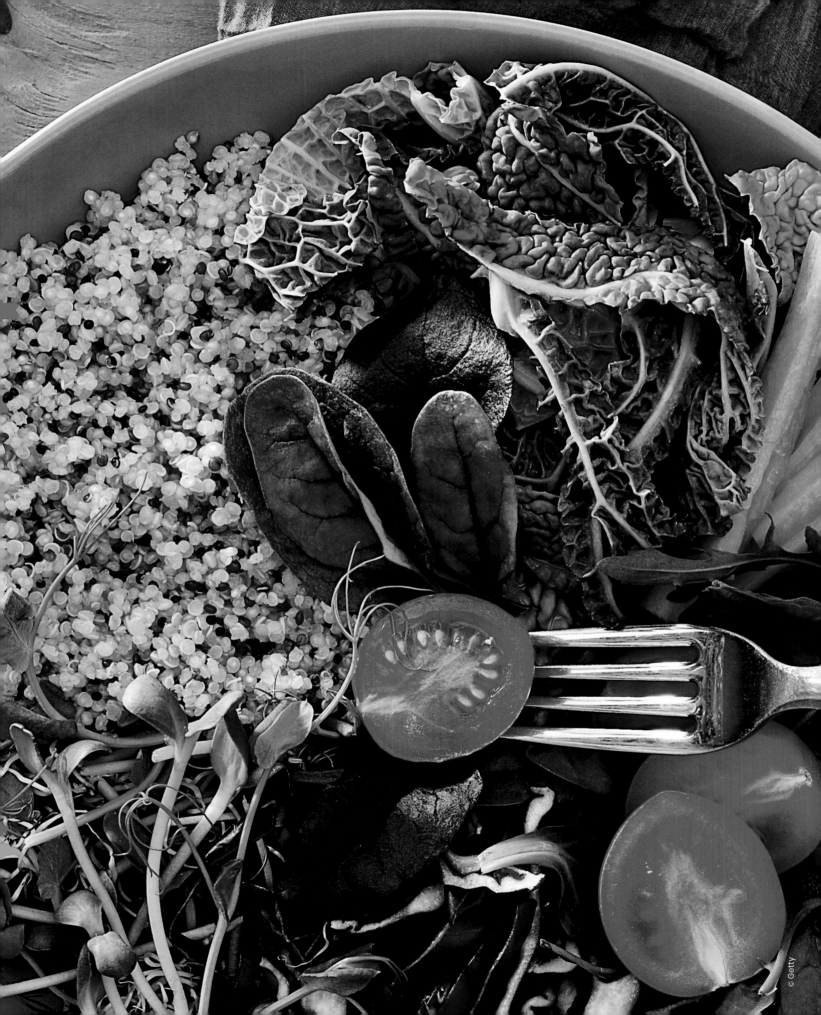

When it comes to chronic inflammation, there is no single cause, but what you choose to eat can have a large impact on the level of inflammation in your body. Some foods in the modern diet have been shown to increase inflammation, particularly those that are ultra-processed, high in sugar and fat, and low in nutritional value.

These types of foods can also lead to weight gain, when eaten to excess, and being overweight can be another contributory factor towards chronic inflammation. Choosing to eat foods that support your body and reduce inflammation can also help you to maintain a healthy weight, though it is not specifically a weight-loss diet. Many of these foods cause a rise in your blood sugar (or glucose) levels; some studies have found a link between high blood sugar and inflammation. Inflammation may also make our cells insulin resistant, which can further increase blood sugar levels.

The anti-inflammatory diet isn't a strict plan or a prescribed protocol; it's simply a term used to describe a way of eating that includes plenty of foods to promote lower levels of chronic inflammation, while reducing the intake of inflammatory foods. An anti-inflammatory way of eating overlaps with other common diets, most significantly the Mediterranean diet. It can be adapted for those who eat animal products, as well as vegetarian and plant-based diets.

We'll go into more detail later, but in short, the aim of the diet is to eat foods that are nutrient dense, minimally processed and packed with antioxidants. It's also important to get a good balance of protein, carbs and healthy fats. Getting enough fibre can also help to reduce inflammation – guidelines suggest we should aim for 30g per day, but the average intake is closer to 20g.

Eating in an anti-inflammatory way isn't complex or expensive. Fruits and vegetables have a starring role, so the aim is to try to get a good variety across each day and week. Dark, leafy, green

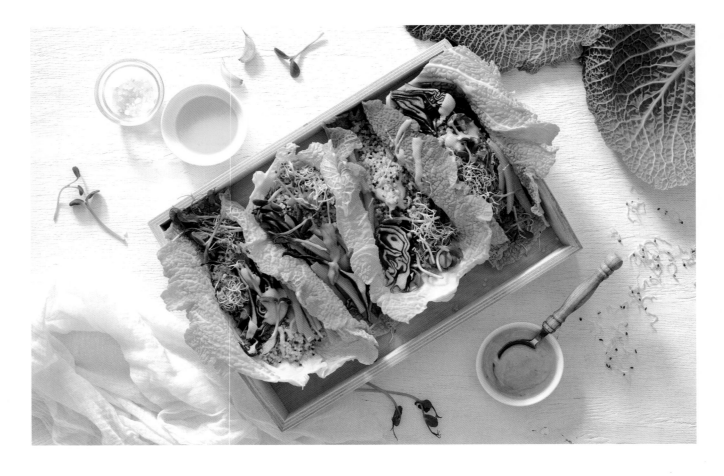

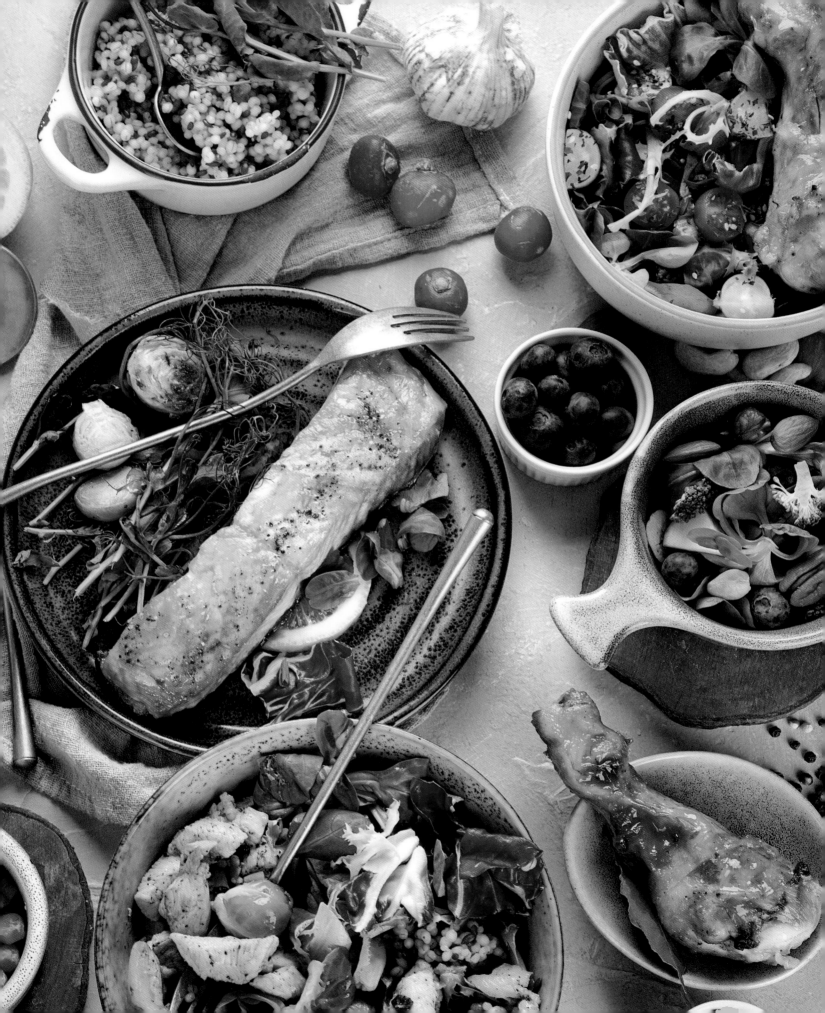

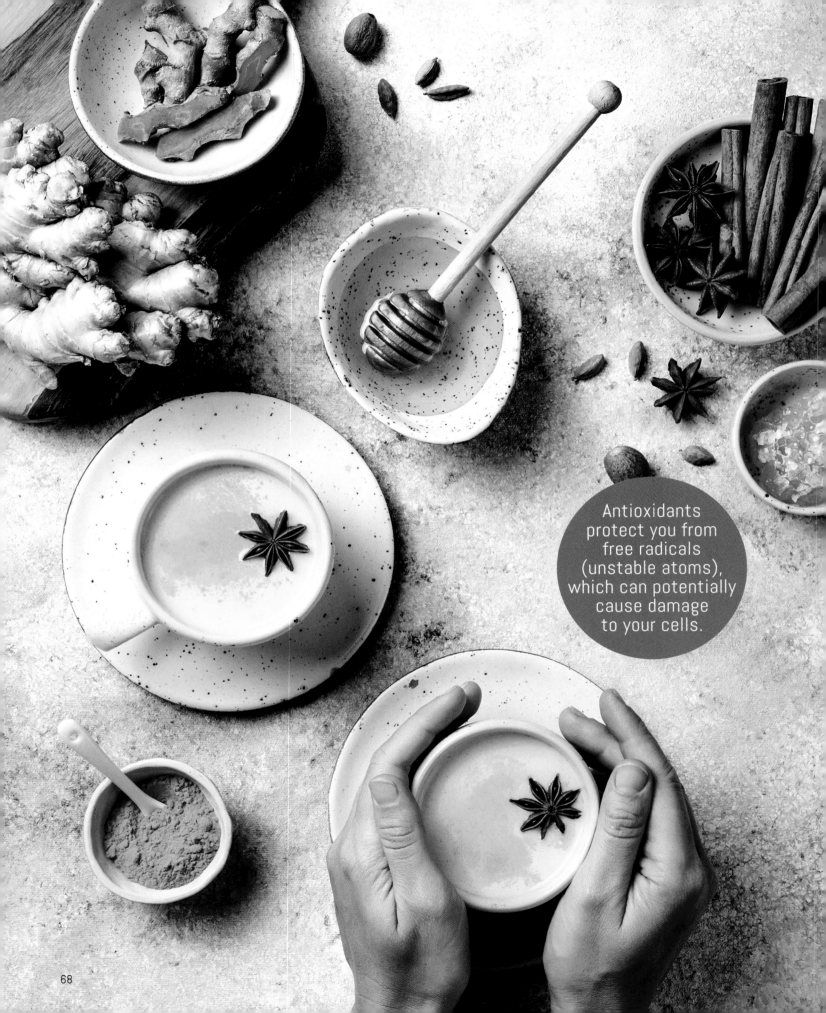

Antioxidants protect you from free radicals (unstable atoms), which can potentially cause damage to your cells.

and cruciferous vegetables, as well as deep-coloured berries and other fruits, are good for being high in antioxidants. To this base you can add healthy fats, such as olive oil or avocado oil, fatty fish like salmon and mackerel, and a mix of nuts and seeds. Some spices are thought to help reduce inflammation in the body, for example turmeric and cinnamon, so consider adding these to your meals.

It's also important to stay hydrated, and there is nothing better than good old water! Water helps to flush any irritants out of your body by helping the body perform its normal elimination procedures – urine is part of our natural filtration system for removing waste products and toxins. Adequate water intake will also help to reduce inflammation in the body.

We know that gut health is intrinsically linked to our immune system and health, so it's not surprising that looking after your gut will help with inflammation. Feed your body with prebiotic and probiotic foods to help support a varied and diverse microbiome. This means including foods that are fermented, like yogurt, sauerkraut or kimchi, or using a supplement.

Over the following pages, we'll be looking at common inflammatory foods and what you could swap them for instead. We'll focus on the specific foods you should include in your diet as much as possible, which will hopefully inspire you to try new foods, cook different meals, and embrace a new anti-inflammatory lifestyle.

Anti-inflammatory food pyramid

A quick and easy guide to the foods that make up a balanced, anti-inflammatory diet, and how much of them you should eat

This diagram gives a great basic overview of what an anti-inflammatory diet looks like. The aim is to consume more of the foods at the bottom of the pyramid and less of those near the top. It can be adapted to suit your dietary preferences (for example, whether to include animal protein and dairy products). At the base of the pyramid are fruits and vegetables, which should form the basis of most meals. Then you have whole grains, followed by healthy fats and oily fish, lean protein sources, spices and herbs, some dairy (or alternatives) and teas. At the top of the pyramid are things like chocolate, sweets and cakes, which can be included in a minimal way as part of a balanced diet.

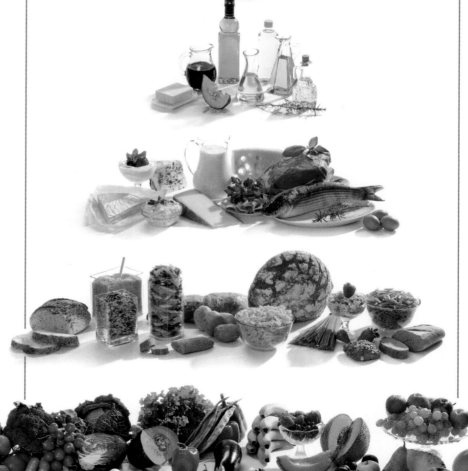

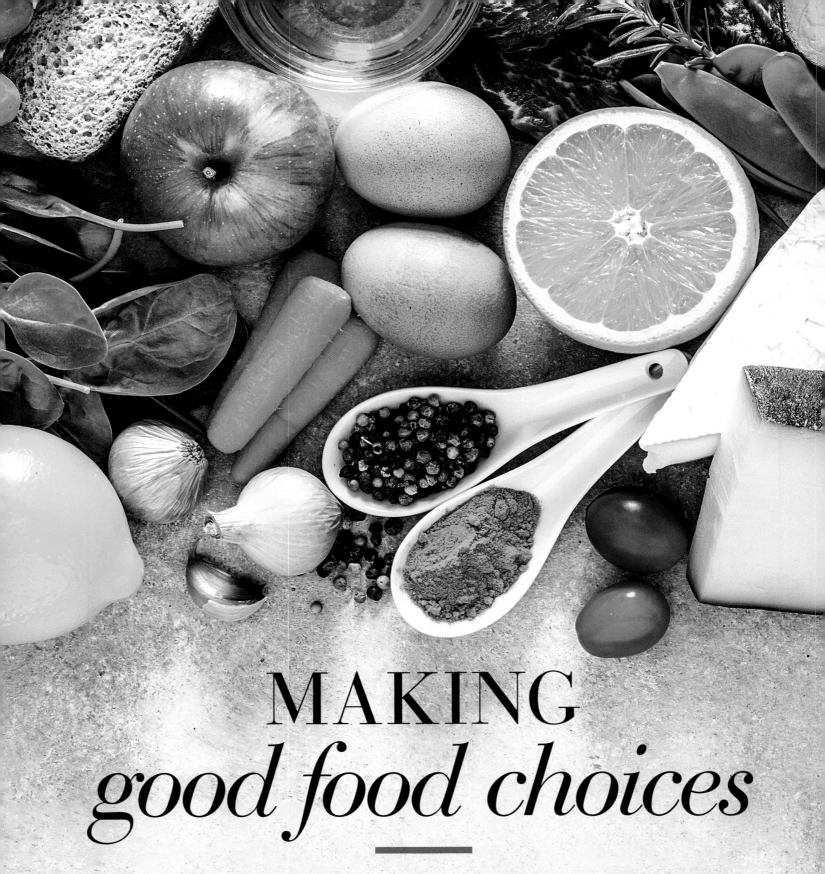

MAKING
good food choices

How to pick the best foods for your lifestyle, budget
and health goals for an anti-inflammatory diet

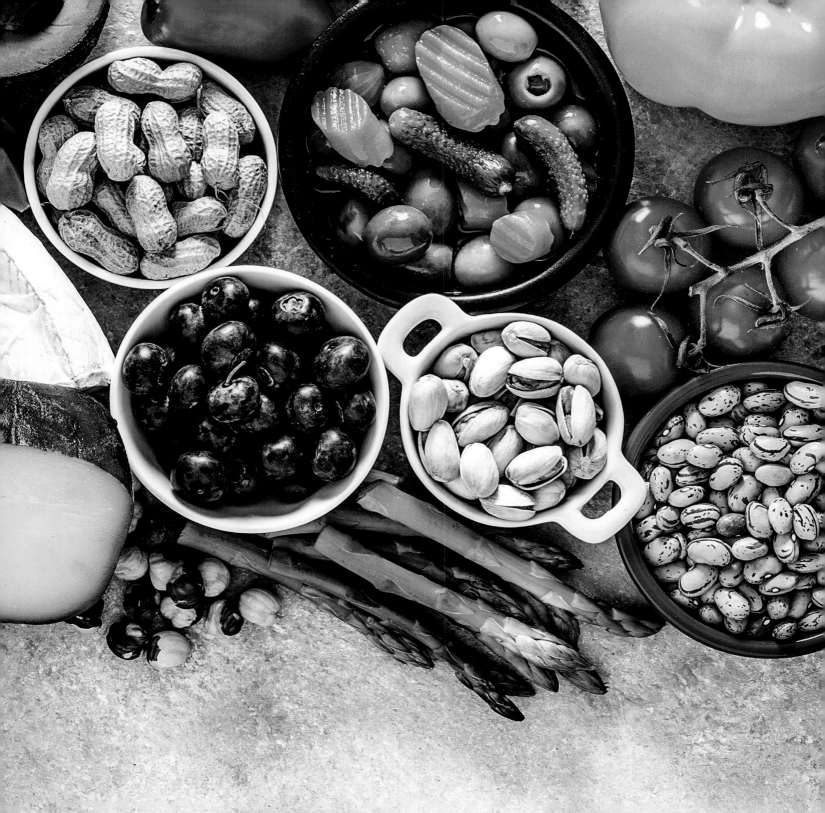

Eating to reduce inflammation in your body isn't just about what foods you eat, but also the quality of the foods. Everyone will be coming at an anti-inflammation diet from a different place, so the focus is on making the best food choices for you, your lifestyle and your budget. Here we will give you some advice around making good food choices, so you can pick and mix what works best for you.

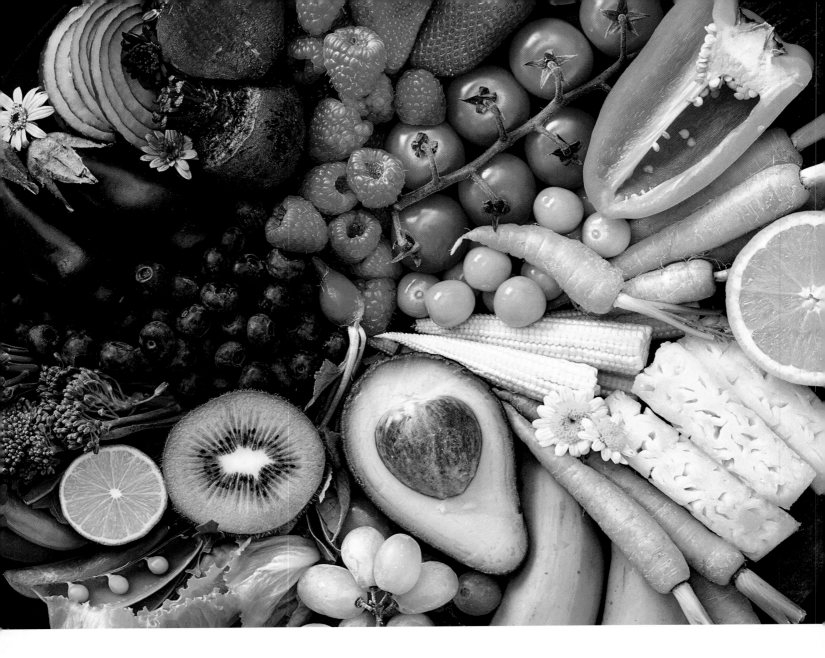

FRUITS AND VEGETABLES – *is fresh and organic best?*

As far as possible, fresh wholefoods are best for an anti-inflammatory diet. So, try to get your fruits and vegetables fresh whenever you can.

If you can go shopping in person to a supermarket or grocer's market, then you can look for the best quality fruits and vegetables you can find. Try to select as wide a variety of fruit and veg as you can, looking to fill your basket with all the colours of the rainbow.

One question that often crops up is whether to buy organic or not. You don't have to buy all your fruits and vegetables organic – this isn't affordable for everyone – but if you can buy some, then this can be very beneficial.

There is the so-called 'Dirty Dozen', which are the foods that are the best ones to try to buy organic, as they tend to have the most residue from pesticides when conventionally grown. This list includes some greens,

apples and pears, nectarines and peaches, grapes, berries, peppers and green beans.

Then there are also the 'Clean 15' fruits and vegetables, which can be more safely bought as non-organic produce. You can see both these lists in full in our boxouts. If you can afford to buy some of your produce organic, then try to prioritise those on the Dirty Dozen list.

Organic produce is produced without any chemicals, using

The Dirty Dozen

Discover the 12 fruits and vegetables that are best to try to buy organic

A new Dirty Dozen list is released every year, showing the most polluted fruits and vegetables. These are the ones you should try to buy organic, listed from most polluted to least. The produce is tested for the list after it has been bought in the supermarket, brought home and washed. It might not be possible for you to buy all of these foods in their organic form, as they are generally more expensive. But if you have the capacity to buy some organic produce, start from the top of the list and work your way down. You can often get organic frozen versions of these products too, which can be cheaper and last longer. Here is the list from 2023:

The additional antioxidants found in organic fruit and veg are equivalent to eating 1-2 extra portions a day!

 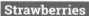
Strawberries

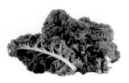
Kale, collard & mustard greens

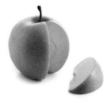
Apples

Cherries

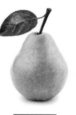
Pears

Blueberries

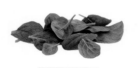
Spinach

Nectarines

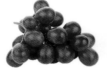
Grapes

Peaches

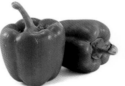
Bell peppers (capsicum)

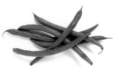
Green beans

natural fertilisers only, unlike more conventional growing techniques. While the levels of pesticides on our foods is relatively low anyway, organic farming has other benefits over intensive farming when it comes to an anti-inflammatory diet. One study in 2014* found that organic crops and crop-based foods (like bread) have up to 60% more key antioxidants than conventionally grown crops – great news for fighting inflammation!

However, it's still much better to buy standard fruit and vegetables than not to buy them at all. If the budget is tight, then shop around and you're sure to find some great deals. Many low-cost supermarkets now offer a selection of fruit and vegetables cheaply each week, changing the varieties on offer regularly. Just don't forget to wash your fruits and vegetables before eating them, as this can remove some traces of pesticides that may have been left on them.

In our busy modern world, it isn't always possible to go to the shops regularly in person, and many of us rely on convenience foods or shopping deliveries to fit around our work and family life. It's perfectly fine to include things like frozen fruits and vegetables, or tinned options, if this is cheaper or easier for you. Again, it's better to include these products than not.

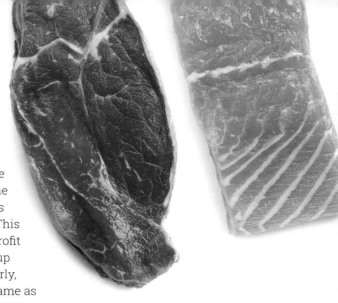

The Clean 15

The fruit and veg that are safest to buy and consume in their non-organic state

Using the same metrics as the Dirty Dozen, there is also a Clean 15 list. These are foods that are still conventionally produced and have the lowest amount of pesticides or residue when bought from the shop. These are fruits and vegetables that you can make good savings on by buying the normal, non-organic versions to help keep to your budget. This list is produced by the non-profit Environmental Working Group (ewg.org), and is updated yearly, though it stays broadly the same as a guide. Here is the list from 2023:

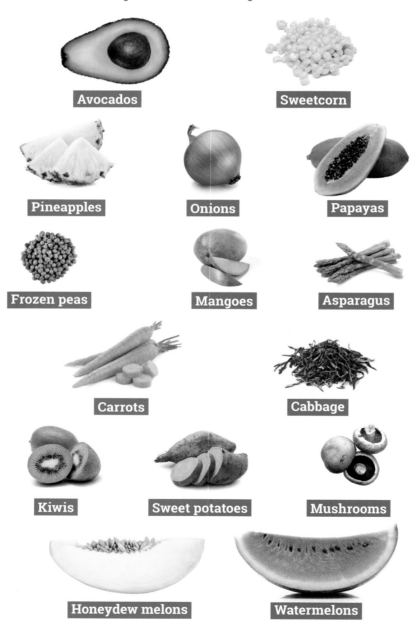

Avocados

Sweetcorn

Pineapples

Onions

Papayas

Frozen peas

Mangoes

Asparagus

Carrots

Cabbage

Kiwis

Sweet potatoes

Mushrooms

Honeydew melons

Watermelons

PICKING YOUR PROTEIN

If you are a meat or fish eater, then again it's about making the best choices that you can for your budget. When you're shopping for meat to include in your diet, try to look for high-quality, grass-fed meat, rather than factory-farmed meat. In this case, it's better to reduce the amount of meat you eat to include high-quality meats when you do eat it, rather than opt for cheaper, processed alternatives.

Organic meat is a good source of omega-3 fatty acids, which is great for those who don't eat fish. Organic, grass-fed meat has around 47% more omega-3 fatty acids than factory-farmed meat, according to the same study we mentioned earlier. It also has higher levels of polyunsaturated fat, higher nutrient levels, and lower saturated fat. If you're looking to reduce inflammation in your body, while including animal protein, then the quality of the food you choose really can make a big difference. If you can, use your local farm shop

*Higher antioxidant and lower cadmium concentrations and lower incidence of pesticide residues in organically grown crops: a systematic literature review and meta-analyses, July 2014

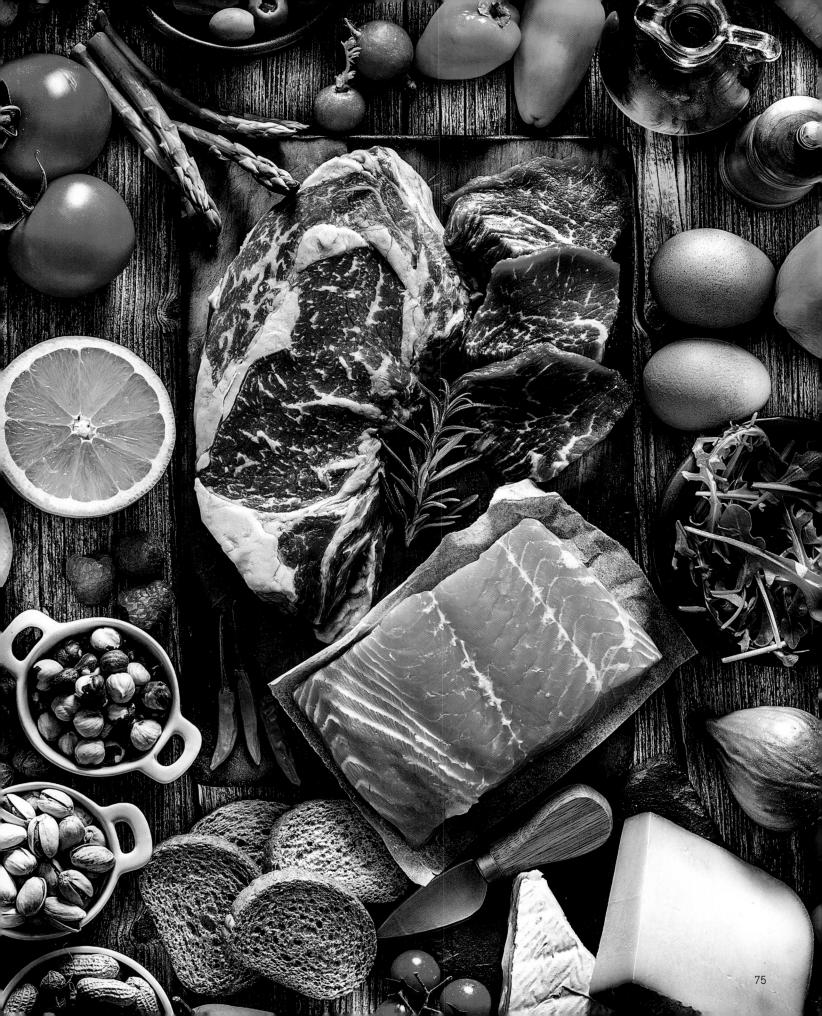

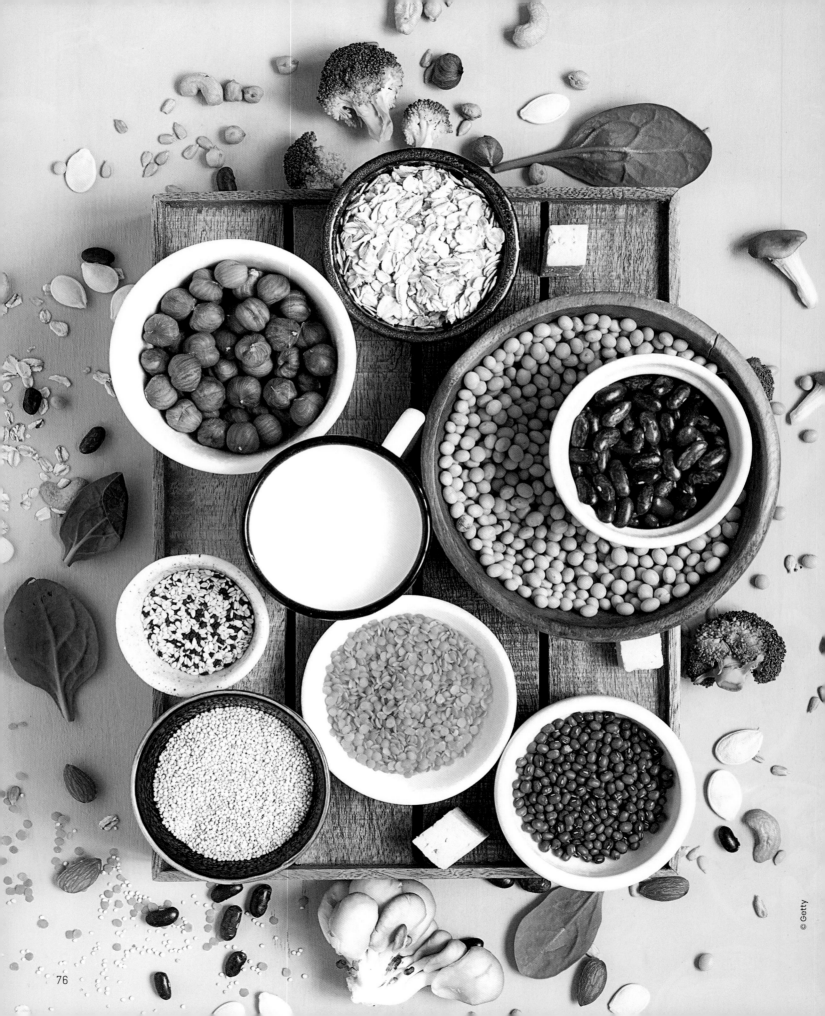

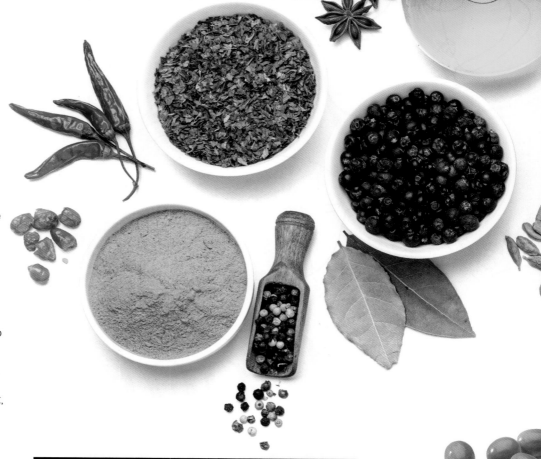

or butcher's shop to buy locally produced meat that is fresh. You can opt for cheaper, less popular cuts to keep the budget down – speak to the butcher who can recommend some nutritious cuts you may not have considered before.

The same is true of fish – wild-caught fish has health properties above factory-raised fish. Salmon is a good example of this. Wild-caught salmon has more nutrients, and a better ratio of omega-3 to omega-6 fats, increasing its anti-inflammatory properties. Wild-caught salmon is also better for the environment, so it's win-win all round! Eggs are the same – organic eggs typically have higher levels of omega-3 fatty acids than non-organic eggs. Given that omega-3 plays a role in reducing inflammation in the body (see our nutrients section for more on this), you can see why opting for free-range and organic protein is worthwhile.

If you follow a vegetarian, vegan or plant-based diet (or any variation within that), animal protein isn't going to be an option. Soybeans are a high-quality protein option, packed with nutrients. It's best to buy soy products as minimally processed as possible. Many of the 'fake meat' products you see are made with soy, but they are highly processed and not the most healthful choice when looking to eat in an anti-inflammatory way. Instead, try soy products like tofu or tempeh, or include edamame beans. This way you're getting all the benefits of the protein and nutrients, without the heavy processing.

WHAT ELSE TO LOOK FOR

Once you've got your protein source and your fruits and vegetables sorted, you then need to consider your other food choices to build a balanced, healthy meal. The aim of an anti-inflammatory diet is to eat foods that are very rich in nutrients, full of antioxidants and also some healthy fats.

Many people worry about the cost of adding new foods into their diet, but you can eat in an anti-inflammatory way without breaking the budget. Getting fermented foods into your diet can increase the healthy bacteria in your gut, which in turn reduces inflammation. These foods can be expensive when you look in the supermarket, but most of them can be made cheaply at home – so when it comes to making good food choices, don't buy the jarred, pre-made versions, and spend a little time in the kitchen instead. For example, sauerkraut is low in calories and high in nutrients. Buying a small jar of it can seem very pricey, but cabbage is cheap to buy and then you only need some sea salt crystals and herbs/spices, plus a little time, to make your own batch.

Many anti-inflammatory grains, legumes and healthy fat sources can be bought cheaply too, especially if you buy in bulk: look for nuts and seeds, a variety of beans and whole grains.

The key thing is to do the best you can. Buy the best quality you can afford. It's better to increase the nutrient-rich food in your diet regardless of where it comes from, and reduce the amount of processed food as far as reasonably possible. By making these good food choices, you can improve your health and reduce inflammation.

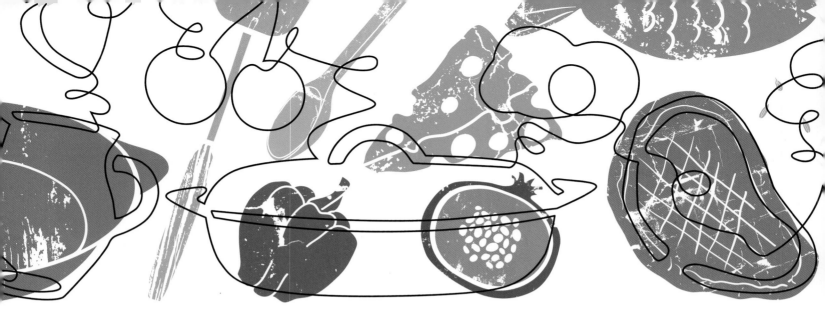

Cooking
METHODS
TO REDUCE INFLAMMATION

**The way you cook your food can make a difference
to the inflammation caused in your body.
We explore the best (and worst) cooking methods**

Knowing what you should be eating to help reduce inflammation is one part of the puzzle, but the way you cook your food can make a big difference too. Some cooking methods will destroy the nutrients in your food, whereas others will help to keep all the goodness in as far as possible.

The best methods for cooking are those that are considered 'gentle', keeping the foods you're cooking as intact as possible. Some foods are also better suited to different cooking methods than other foods. Many foods are susceptible to damage when cooked at a high heat, which means things like frying, using the barbeque, grill or roasting in hot oil can break down some of the nutrients. Using a microwave is not ideal; despite being highly convenient, the short burst of very high heat can zap those nutrients.

That's not to say you can never use these methods. Grilling is a great option for things like fish or vegetable skewers, as they don't need to be cooked for very long, so they're not exposed to the high heat for vast lengths of time. Meats, however, need to be cooked for longer, losing many nutrients along the way. Not only that, when meat is cooked using a high-temperature method, it can cause the formation of heterocyclic amines (HCA), which

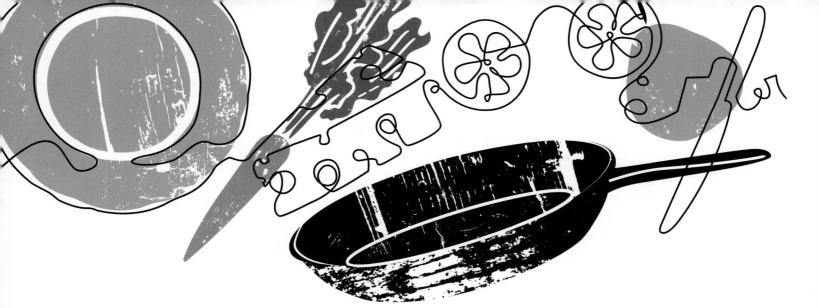

can contribute to inflammation, and other changes in the body.

In general, frying isn't an ideal cooking method due to the amount of oil needed as well as the cooking temperatures involved. However, stir frying is a bit different and can be a good way to quickly cook food with little to no oil – as long as you have a good pan. As you keep the food moving around the pan as it's cooking, you're helping it to cook much quicker and retain all those nutrients, especially in your vegetables.

If you're looking to reduce inflammation in your body, the key to cooking your food is to use lower temperatures and add moisture. Steaming is a great way to cook, as it's very gentle to the food and doesn't need any added oil. A steamer pot keeps the food out of the water, allowing the hot steam to circulate and cook the food. This is a great way to do your vegetables – they don't need long, so keep an eye on them and make sure they don't overcook and become soggy.

When it comes to your meat, why not try poaching? Again, no oil is needed and it doesn't expose the meat to very high temperatures. You can poach in water or stock, and add herbs and spices to your water base to infuse added flavour. Poaching heats the meat very carefully and gently, retaining all the nutrients.

Don't worry, the oven isn't off limits. Baking is a convenient cooking method, and it can be very healthful as long as you're not adding lots of oil and heating the food very high. It's best to use the middle of the oven, so there's room for the hot air to circulate around the oven space. Again, adding moisture can help, which can be as simple as adding vegetables to the bottom of your cooking dish and adding protein on top, away from the base of the dish.

You can adapt your cooking methods to what you have available and what fits in to your lifestyle. It's just about being mindful around how you cook, and taking the time to prepare and cook gently when you can.

> Add inflammation-reducing spices to your food during cooking to add extra benefits with minimal effort.

EATING RAW FOODS

Sometimes you don't need to cook at all! Eating some raw foods can be beneficial on an anti-inflammatory diet as they are full of goodness. Having a salad on the side of your dinner plate, for example, is a quick way to add extra nutrients to your meal – try to vary the salad vegetables you use to include a wide variety, such as lettuce, spinach, radish, carrot, avocado, cucumber, peppers, and so on. Increase the benefits by adding a drizzle of good-quality extra virgin olive oil and some lemon juice as a dressing. If you have a snack during the day, there is no need to cook anything – opt for a piece of fruit, nuts and seeds, or crudités with hummus. You can try to introduce a few raw vegetables that you might not have considered too, such as kale, which can be eaten in a salad or thrown into a smoothie. It's also good to add some gut-boosting foods, such as sauerkraut and kimchi, to your meals.

Common
INFLAMMATORY
FOODS

If you're looking to reduce inflammation in your body, these are the most common culprits

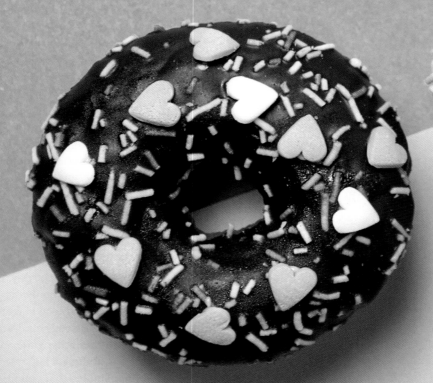

There are essentially two parts to an anti-inflammatory diet. First is knowing what foods to add into your diet that have an anti-inflammatory effect. Second is knowing what foods to remove from your diet that may contribute to inflammation.

Over the next few pages, we'll look at the most common foods that have been shown to cause inflammation so that you can begin to eat in a way that supports your health. It might not be possible or desirable to remove all these foods at once, but even cutting down or starting with one food type can have a beneficial result.

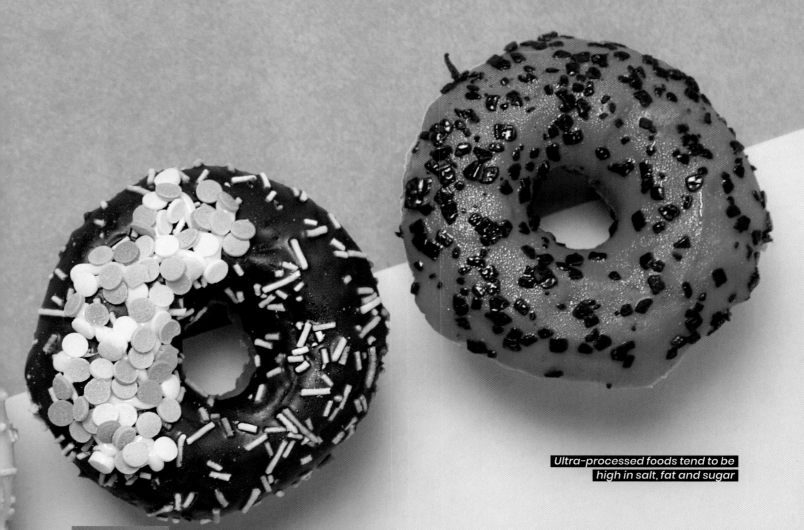

ULTRA-PROCESSED FOODS

Some chronic inflammation can be linked to a high intake of ultra-processed foods. These are foods that go through multiple processes to produce, and include ingredients that you might not recognise and certainly wouldn't have access to in a typical home kitchen. These foods are designed and manufactured to taste a certain way and also to last a long time on the shelf. They are far removed from natural wholefoods, and retain little goodness or nutrients. They often have to have vitamins and minerals added back in to give them any healthful properties. If you look at the ingredients list on the packaging, you might notice that they have additives, colouring and preservatives.

Unfortunately, the typical Western diet is packed with ultra-processed foods. In a 2018 study* looking at ultra-processed food consumption in the UK, the most commonly eaten foods in this category were industrialised bread, pre-packaged meals, breakfast cereals and sausages/reconstituted meat products. This category of foods also includes things like cakes, biscuits, sweets and pastries, as well as baked beans, tinned soup and meat alternatives. All of these foods are far removed from any of the original wholefood ingredients. According to the same study, up to 56% of calories in a typical UK diet come from ultra-processed food sources. While this study looked at UK diets, many other Western countries, including the United States and elsewhere in Europe, have similar statistics.

These ultra-processed foods are often high in salt, fat and sugar, and typically have a long list of ingredients. If you're looking to start an anti-inflammatory diet, then reducing or eliminating your intake of ultra-processed foods is a great place to start, and can have an immediate impact on your health.

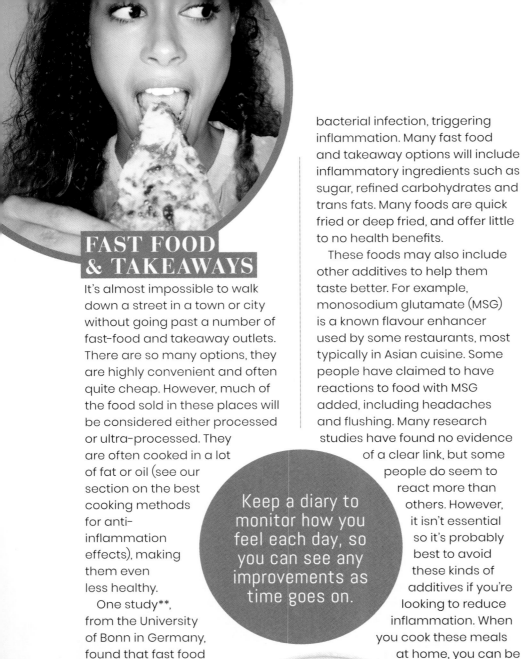

FAST FOOD & TAKEAWAYS

It's almost impossible to walk down a street in a town or city without going past a number of fast-food and takeaway outlets. There are so many options, they are highly convenient and often quite cheap. However, much of the food sold in these places will be considered either processed or ultra-processed. They are often cooked in a lot of fat or oil (see our section on the best cooking methods for anti-inflammation effects), making them even less healthy.

One study**, from the University of Bonn in Germany, found that fast food can cause an immune response in the body in the same way as it would for a bacterial infection, triggering inflammation. Many fast food and takeaway options will include inflammatory ingredients such as sugar, refined carbohydrates and trans fats. Many foods are quick fried or deep fried, and offer little to no health benefits.

These foods may also include other additives to help them taste better. For example, monosodium glutamate (MSG) is a known flavour enhancer used by some restaurants, most typically in Asian cuisine. Some people have claimed to have reactions to food with MSG added, including headaches and flushing. Many research studies have found no evidence of a clear link, but some people do seem to react more than others. However, it isn't essential so it's probably best to avoid these kinds of additives if you're looking to reduce inflammation. When you cook these meals at home, you can be sure of what is going into each dish.

Keep a diary to monitor how you feel each day, so you can see any improvements as time goes on.

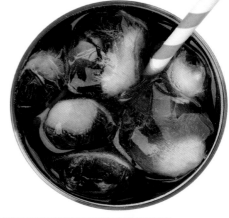

ARTIFICIAL & ADDED SUGARS

It's probably no surprise that sugar isn't great for your body. We already know that too much sugar is bad for your teeth, can make it harder to maintain a healthy weight, and is a contributory factor towards diseases like type 2 diabetes. However, too much sugar can also cause an inflammatory response in your body.

Processed foods tend to have a lot of sugar in them. It helps with the taste, texture and longevity of the products. If you're trying to reduce inflammation in your body, then it's worth cutting down on these processed foods, as mentioned earlier. This means things like soft drinks, pastries, chocolate, sweets, cakes, biscuits and ready meals. Added sugars can sometimes be hidden under a different name, such as fructose, corn syrup, sucrose, maltose and so on, so it's worth

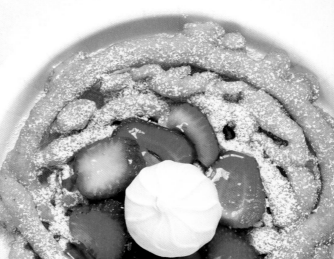

getting to grips with reading ingredient labels. You might be surprised to learn which foods have sugar added to them – many stock powders or cubes do, packaged breads often have sugar in them, and breakfast cereals can be high in sugars, too.

Where possible, choose low-sugar foods, or stick to natural sugars like honey in small quantities. It's fine to eat whole fruits, even though they have a lot of natural sugars in them, as they are a good source of antioxidants and fibre.

COOKING OILS

Cooking oils are an essential in the kitchen, but not all oils are made equal. Cheap vegetable oils have been used for decades and yet these are often high in omega-6 fatty acids and low in omega-3. It's thought that a diet that is unbalanced in omega-6 and omega-3 can lead to inflammation and disease. High levels of omega-6 are often found in these less healthy unsaturated fats; though we do want some omega-6 in our diet, it's much better to get it from natural plant sources and to ensure a good balance with

> " Where possible, choose low-sugar foods, or stick to natural sugars like honey in small quantities

higher levels of omega-3.

Those oils that are highest in omega-6 include things like canola oil, sunflower oil, corn oil and soybean oil. These are oils that are often used in processed and fast food, as they are cheap and easy to get hold of – another reason to avoid convenience and ultra-processed foods! When you're cooking at home, you can have more control over your choice of cooking oil – opt for things like extra-virgin olive oil, perfect for baking, drizzling and medium-temperature cooking; or avocado oil, which is better for higher-heat cooking methods, as it has a higher smoke point.

ALCOHOL

Drinking too much alcohol has been linked to increased inflammation. It can impact on your gut health, which in itself may cause, or prevent the repair of, inflammation around the body. Excessive alcohol consumption can prevent the liver from doing its job properly, detoxing your system, which again can increase the chance of inflammation. Essentially, alcohol can both cause inflammation and prevent the body from regulating inflammation. It does very much depend on how much you drink, and every person is different in what they can tolerate, but generally speaking, less is more when it comes to alcohol. There are some studies that suggest a glass of red wine can have an antioxidant effect, but non-alcoholic options are more beneficial overall. If you do drink, try to limit yourself to one or two glasses at a time and always have alcohol-free days in between to allow the body to recover and repair.

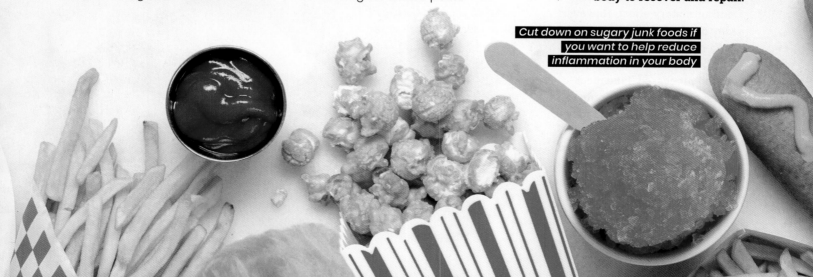

Cut down on sugary junk foods if you want to help reduce inflammation in your body

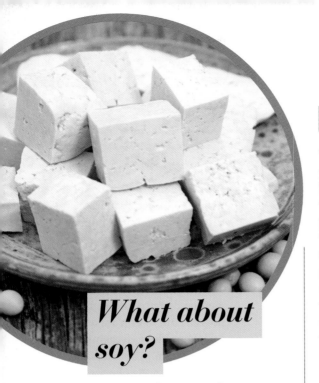

What about soy?

Soy is one of those products that has been quite contentious in recent years. It was, for a long time, thought to be quite inflammatory and even linked to certain types of cancer. However, this has been widely debunked and now it's thought that soy might actually have an anti-inflammatory effect and actually protect against some cancers. Soy is more widely eaten in Eastern countries; one study of more than a thousand Chinese women (Shanghai Women's Health Study) found that the more soy products women consumed, the less inflammation they experienced. Soy is high in omega-3 fatty acids, which have an anti-inflammatory effect. However, soy can be heavily processed and this can remove a lot of the benefits. So, those soy-based processed 'fake meat' meal options are not going to support your health and may increase inflammation due to the heavy processing involved. But more natural soy products, like tofu, miso or tempeh, can have health benefits.

© Getty

SOME MEATS

You don't need to eat a plant-based diet to reduce inflammation, unless you want to. But some meat and animal protein can be a contributory factor towards inflammation. One of the worst culprits is processed and reconstituted meats. This includes anything that has been cured, smoked, salted or fermented. These types of meats are high in saturated fat and are highly processed, which can cause inflammation. High amounts of processed meat have also been linked to a larger risk of bowel cancer, according to the World Cancer Research Fund. This can be due to chemicals that are found in these meats naturally, added during processing, or produced during the cooking process. Processed meats to avoid include ham, bacon, salami, hot dogs, pepperoni and sausages – it is best to eliminate these as fully from your diet as possible, as there is no prescribed safe limit.

It's also a good idea to cut down on red meat, which includes all fresh, minced or frozen beef, pork and lamb. These meats have also been linked to inflammation when eaten too often. If you do want to keep red meat in your diet, then try to opt for the best quality that you can afford. Grass-fed, organic meat a couple of times a week is far better for your health than cheaper, industrially farmed meat on a daily basis.

It's fine to keep poultry and fish on your plate as animal proteins if that suits your dietary preferences, but commercially produced meat can contribute to inflammation. Animals that are kept in caged or cramped conditions are not getting a good level of exercise, so are more likely to have excess fat. Not only that, they are not always fed the most natural diet, leading to a poorer-quality end product. Farmed fish can have similar problems, and the nutrition of conventionally farmed eggs is lower, too. Most products in supermarkets are at the lower end of the quality scale, so where possible source your meats, eggs and fish from local suppliers for a high-quality product.

*Ultra-Processed Food Consumption and Chronic Non-Communicable Diseases-Related Dietary Nutrient Profile in the UK (2008–2014), May 2018

> Ease into your diet slowly, and replace one type of inflammatory food at a time rather than all at once.

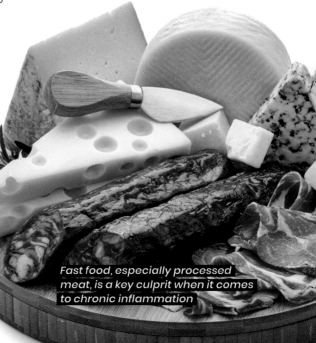

Fast food, especially processed meat, is a key culprit when it comes to chronic inflammation

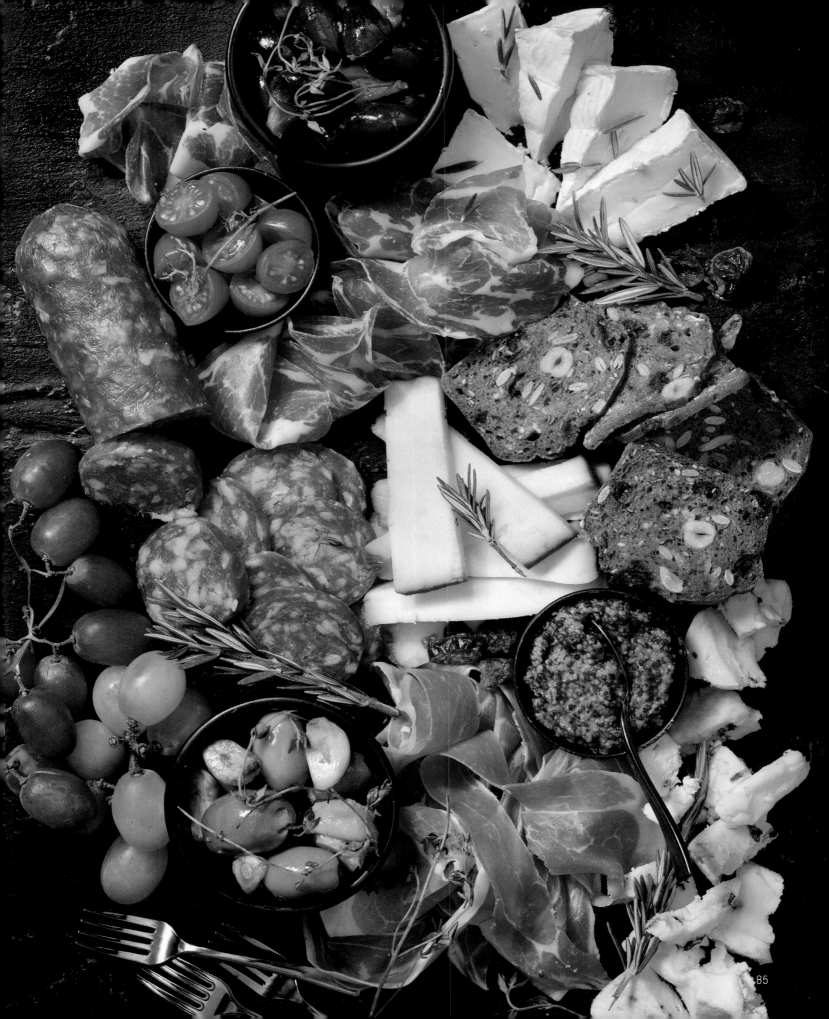

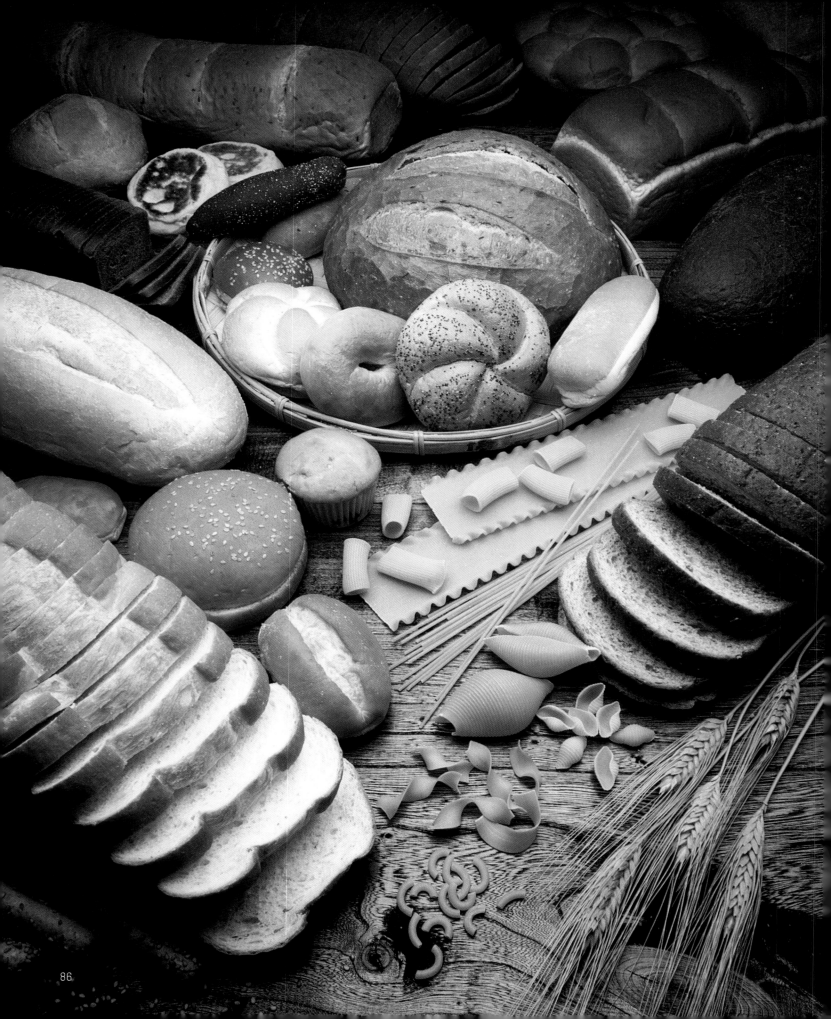

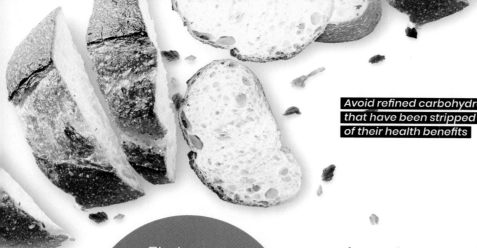

Find some 'fakeaway' recipes to replace fast food so you don't have to miss out on your favourite meals.

DAIRY

Dairy is another food group that can cause an inflammatory response in some people. Dairy products are those that are made from or contain the milk of certain mammals, like cows, sheep or goats. Milk, in particular, is quite a common allergen and many people who are not allergic to it, may be sensitive to it. However, most studies conclude that dairy as a whole group isn't entirely inflammatory, but some products are more likely to cause inflammation than others.

Generally, avoid those made with whole milk or full fat, which includes whole milks, hard cheeses, ice cream, cream, butter and full-fat yogurt. You might find that you can tolerate other forms of dairy, but you may need to experiment and keep a food diary to see if dairy has an impact on the way you feel. There are, fortunately, a lot of good alternatives available now.

REFINED CARBOHYDRATES & GLUTEN

Grains and carbohydrates are a great base for a healthy diet, but refined versions are a different story. Refined grains are stripped of a lot of what makes them healthy, such as the fibre and vitamins. What's left is a processed shell with few nutrients. These refined grains raise your blood-sugar levels when you consume them, which can lead to chronic inflammation if you eat them a lot. They have also been linked to diseases like type 2 diabetes. Common examples of these refined grains and carbohydrates include white bread, white rice, white flour, white pasta and noodles. Refined flour is then also used to make things like biscuits and cakes as well. Popular breakfast cereals are often made with refined grains and can then have things like sugar added to them, making them highly inflammatory.

Ideally you want to eat wholegrains where possible, but unfortunately it's not always as simple as it should be. There is no international definition for what 'wholegrain' means; having it on the packet doesn't mean you're getting the whole of the grain every time. A wholegrain bread in the supermarket, for example, is still highly processed, even if it seems a healthier alternative. It's always better to make at home or buy fresh when you can.

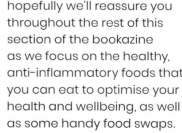

The final word

This can all seem quite overwhelming when looked at as a whole. It might seem like this kind of anti-inflammatory diet is very restrictive and doesn't leave a lot left to eat! But hopefully we'll reassure you throughout the rest of this section of the bookazine as we focus on the healthy, anti-inflammatory foods that you can eat to optimise your health and wellbeing, as well as some handy food swaps.

**Western Diet Triggers NLRP3-Dependent Innate Immune Reprogramming, January 2018

INFLAMMATORY
food swaps

Our handy at-a-glance guide will give you some ideas for swapping out inflammatory foods for better alternatives

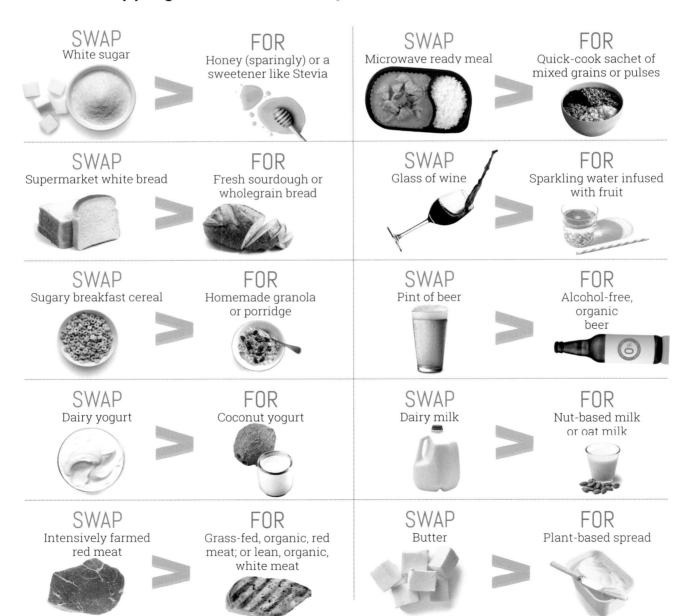

SWAP	FOR	SWAP	FOR
White sugar	Honey (sparingly) or a sweetener like Stevia	Microwave ready meal	Quick-cook sachet of mixed grains or pulses
Supermarket white bread	Fresh sourdough or wholegrain bread	Glass of wine	Sparkling water infused with fruit
Sugary breakfast cereal	Homemade granola or porridge	Pint of beer	Alcohol-free, organic beer
Dairy yogurt	Coconut yogurt	Dairy milk	Nut-based milk or oat milk
Intensively farmed red meat	Grass-fed, organic, red meat; or lean, organic, white meat	Butter	Plant-based spread

© Getty

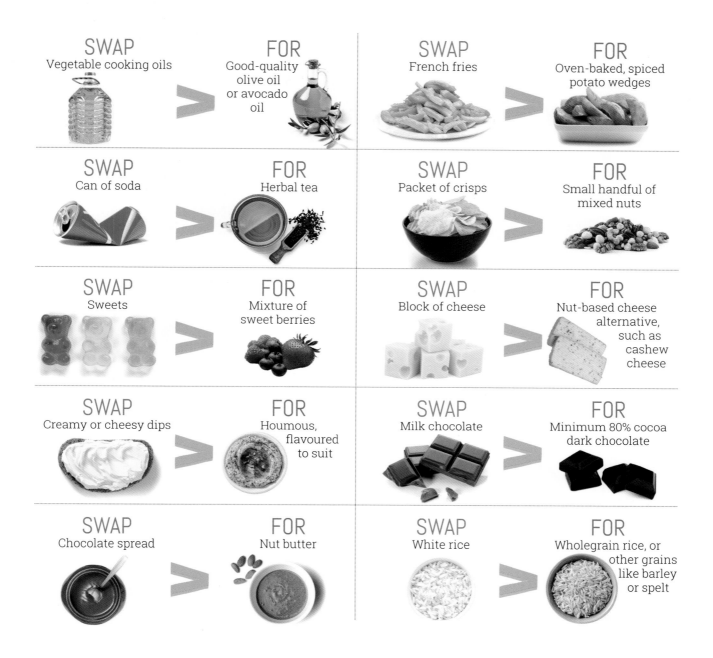

SWAP Vegetable cooking oils > **FOR** Good-quality olive oil or avocado oil	**SWAP** French fries > **FOR** Oven-baked, spiced potato wedges
SWAP Can of soda > **FOR** Herbal tea	**SWAP** Packet of crisps > **FOR** Small handful of mixed nuts
SWAP Sweets > **FOR** Mixture of sweet berries	**SWAP** Block of cheese > **FOR** Nut-based cheese alternative, such as cashew cheese
SWAP Creamy or cheesy dips > **FOR** Houmous, flavoured to suit	**SWAP** Milk chocolate > **FOR** Minimum 80% cocoa dark chocolate
SWAP Chocolate spread > **FOR** Nut butter	**SWAP** White rice > **FOR** Wholegrain rice, or other grains like barley or spelt

Read your packets

You might find a lot of 'healthier' alternatives on the shelves, but when it comes to eating in an anti-inflammatory way, it's worth ditching packaged products entirely. These products can still contain additives, flavourings or ingredients that can contribute to inflammation. Read the packaging – if you must buy something prepared, make sure you understand all the ingredients listed. Most of the food swaps we've suggested can be made quickly and simply. You might need to shop around to find everything you need. There are a number of small businesses that offer things like cheese alternatives that can be much nicer than what's on offer at your local supermarket.

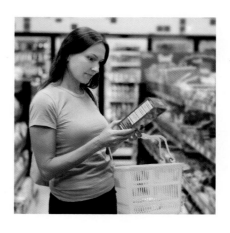

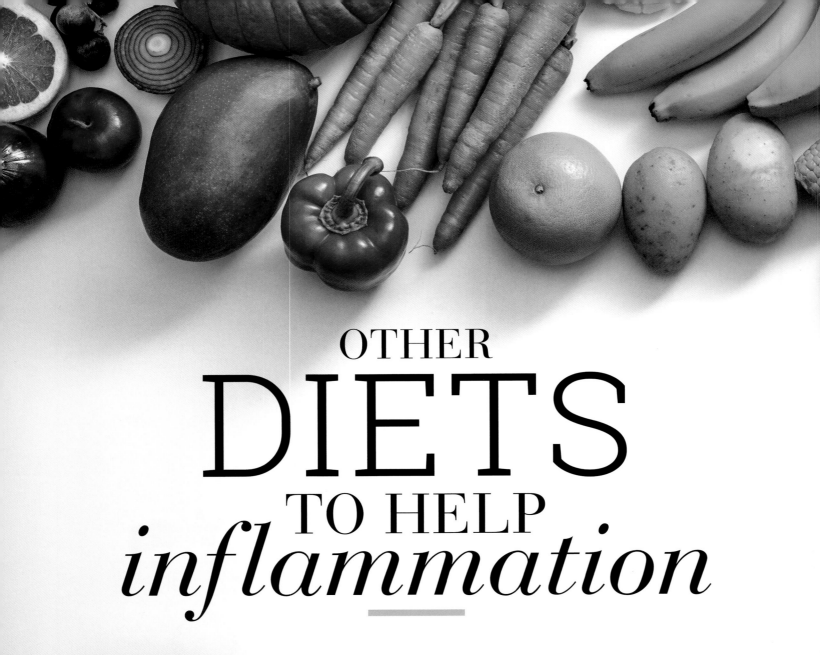

OTHER
DIETS
TO HELP
inflammation

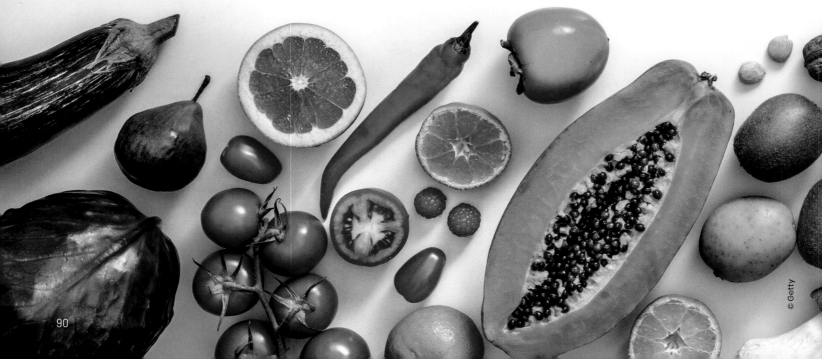

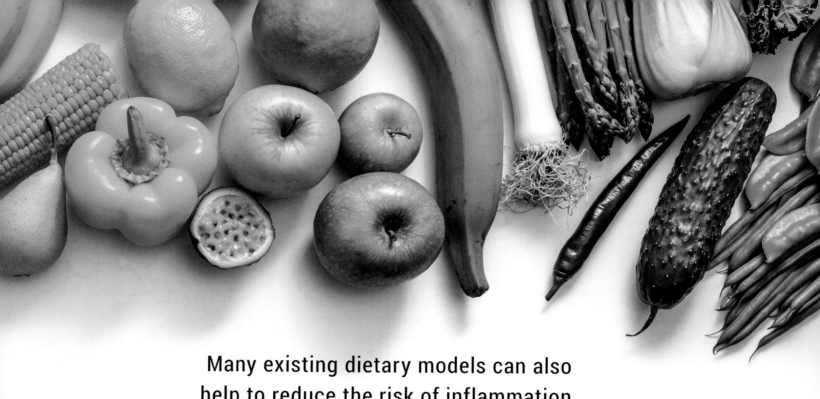

Many existing dietary models can also help to reduce the risk of inflammation. Let's take a look at some of them here

In this book, we've talked about ways in which you can adapt your existing diet to an anti-inflammatory way of eating. However, there are many other diets out there that you can choose to follow, which all help to reduce inflammation because they follow many of the basic principles that we've already discussed in the previous pages.

Here we will look at a few of the most popular diets you might have come across, explain a bit about what they are, and discuss how they can contribute to a reduction in inflammation to help you make an informed decision on what is right for you.

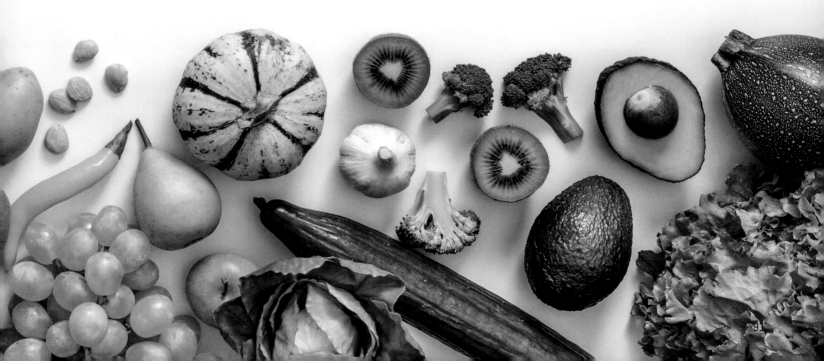

ELIMINATION DIET

Elimination diets are often performed under the supervision of a medical professional to help identify food sensitivities, but you can apply the principles to your own diet to find out if certain foods cause any unwanted reactions in your body.

Sometimes we're sensitive to some foods and this can cause inflammation, whereas we can be fine with others. Following an elimination diet means that you can personalise what you eat more precisely to support your health goals.

This kind of elimination diet fits in nicely with the anti-inflammatory diet we've already discussed in this book, as many of the foods we promote are unlikely to cause sensitivities in the majority of people. But doing an elimination diet can help you discover if things like gluten or dairy are problematic for you.

You do need to be quite organised and disciplined to follow a proper elimination diet. The idea is to remove a particular group of foods from your diet completely for a period of time, and then reintroduce them one at a time. You will need to keep some kind of food diary or symptom tracker so that you can identify which foods you might be sensitive to. If you're sensitive to a food, this can irritate the lining of your gut, causing inflammation, and triggering a range of symptoms from stomach issues to headaches. Sometimes you might not even know you're having symptoms until you remove certain food types, as you could be used to feeling a certain way.

Successful elimination diets can help with a range of symptoms, such as bloating, depression, fatigue or rashes. This is why it's important to make sure you write down everything you feel or notice in your food diary, as the symptoms could be varied. It's also important to remove the foods from your diet long enough so that any traces are gone and symptoms calmed down before you reintroduce any foods – usually this is about three weeks.

The most common food sensitivities that you can identify through this kind of elimination diet includes gluten, eggs, dairy, sugar or sweeteners, and soy. You can opt to eliminate just one food type if you've got a good idea of what might be affecting you, or you can eliminate multiple foods. The more you exclude, the longer the reintroduction stage will take as you need to only bring one food back into your diet at a time so that you can be precise about what is or isn't causing issues. You will need to be careful when reading food labels to ensure you don't accidentally ingest small amounts of the food you are eliminating.

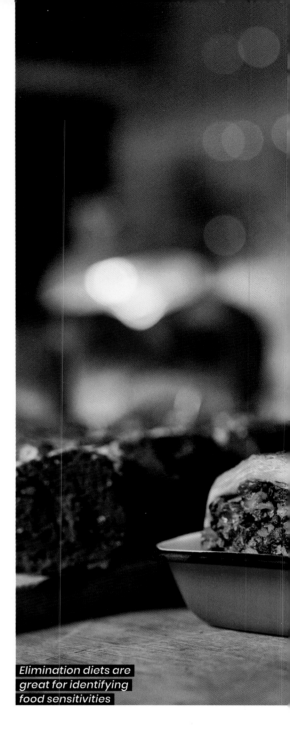

Elimination diets are great for identifying food sensitivities

> Get the whole family involved in meal planning – the mosre support you have, the easier it will be to follow.

MEDITERRANEAN DIET

One of the most popular diets for good health and wellbeing is the Mediterranean diet – and for good reason. This diet is based on the way that people eat in Mediterranean countries and has many health benefits. It can help with your risk of heart

© Getty

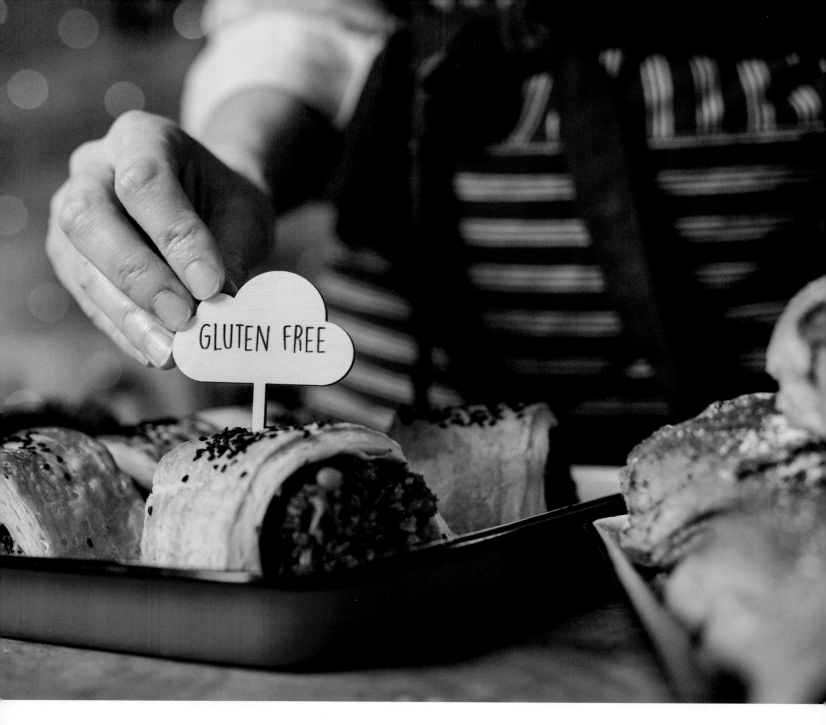

disease, diabetes and chronic illness. It is also naturally anti-inflammatory. Therefore, it's no wonder that doctors around the world are recommending it to their patients.

The typical Mediterranean diet is high in vegetables, fruits, beans, legumes, grains, nuts, and healthy fats and oils. It also includes oily fish, as well as a small amount of meat and dairy products. As such, it is suitable for most people, as it can be easily adapted to eliminate animal products or dairy as required. Most countries will have some version of a recommended healthy diet (for example, the Eatwell Guide in the UK or the Dietary Guidelines for Americans), which are closely linked to the Mediterranean diet, such are its known benefits.

It's no wonder that doctors around the world are recommending it to their patients

The Mediterranean diet is quite well balanced. It doesn't eliminate fats or carbohydrates like many fad diets do. Instead, it focuses on a good balance of all the major food groups to give our body the energy it needs. It's also quite straightforward with few rules to follow. It's a lifestyle change, not a weight-loss diet, which means that it's easier to sustain long term.

It's generally low in saturated fats, but it's not a low-fat diet. The key is picking good, heart-healthy monounsaturated fats like olive oil and nuts. For those who do eat animal products, then it's about having small amounts and the best quality you can afford. It's very rich in fibre too, from the high quantities of wholegrain cereals and grains, vegetables, beans and legumes. We know

that fibre is an important part of gut health and inflammation response. The diet is naturally high in antioxidants, which again is important for managing inflammation, and it's high in nutrients too.

Alcohol can be consumed as part of the Mediterranean diet, but it is in moderation and never to excess. The odd glass of red wine is often enjoyed with

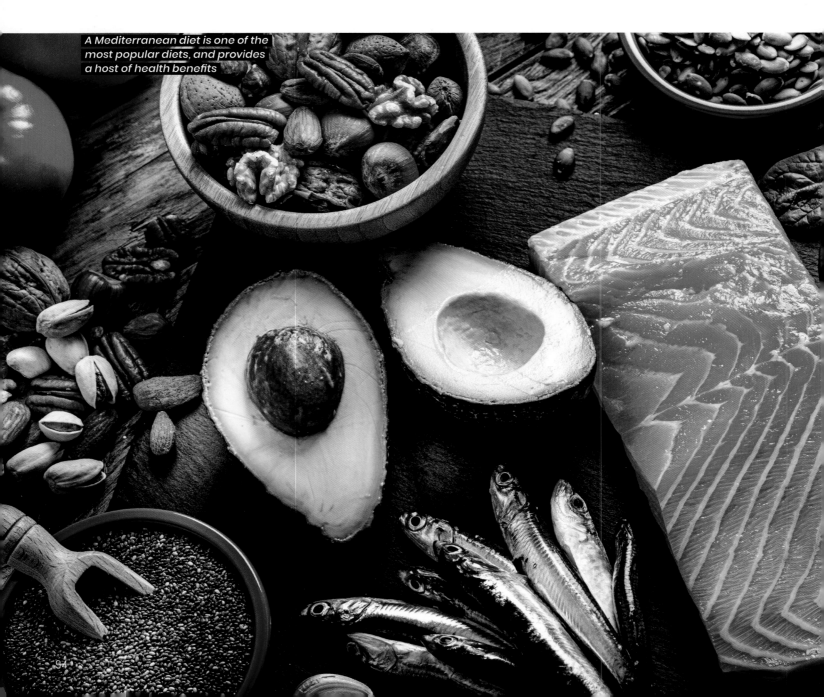

A Mediterranean diet is one of the most popular diets, and provides a host of health benefits

dinner socially. Processed foods are almost entirely eliminated as well, with meals made from simple, basic ingredients, flavoured with natural foods, spices and oils.

As you can see, it's similar to the anti-inflammation diet in many ways, so you can access resources and recipes on the Mediterranean diet to help support your new lifestyle.

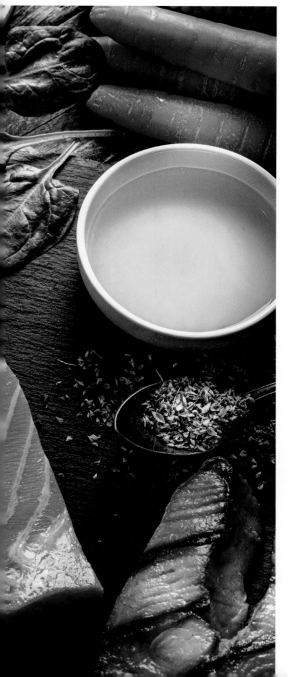

KETO DIETS AND INFLAMMATION

The keto diet has been having a moment of popularity, but is it any good for inflammation? Well, it depends really on what you're eating, and the jury's out. The keto diet is very high in fat, but incredibly low in carbohydrates. It has been used successfully in the control of some chronic illnesses, such as diabetes or epilepsy. However, for the vast majority of people, it's a difficult diet to follow and eliminates many healthy foods that can help with inflammation. Even some fruits and vegetables are considered too high-carb for this diet, and there is quite a reliance on animal protein. The diet does promote choosing good-quality produce, lots of leafy, green vegetables and healthy fat sources, which will all help to reduce inflammation. As with any diet like this, it is possible to do it in a healthy, anti-inflammatory way, and it's also possible to do it while eating a large amount of inflammatory foods. If it's something you're interested in, do your research before embarking on the diet.

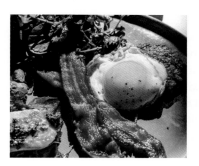

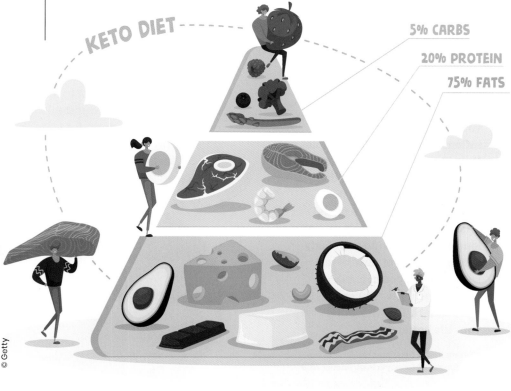

KETO DIET

5% CARBS
20% PROTEIN
75% FATS

© Getty

INTERMITTENT FASTING AND INFLAMMATION

There is some evidence that intermittent fasting can help with inflammation. One study* from 2019 found that fasting improves inflammatory disease. It found that this was due to a reduction in monocytes in the blood, reducing inflammation. It's thought that the benefits come from eating less, as the Western diet often includes more food, more often, than at any time in the past. Therefore, it's not about extreme fasting patterns to gain the benefits. The best and most sustainable way to include intermittent fasting in your lifestyle is to limit your eating to a normal daily window that fits in with your circadian rhythm. You could, for example, pick an eight- hour window that fits in with your lifestyle and eat your main meals within this time only, giving your body the other 16 hours for repair and recovery. Giving your body a break can help your gut, immune system and inflammation. Try, for example, 11am-7pm if you prefer a later breakfast, or 8am-4pm if that fits your life better. You don't have to follow this 16/8 model if that doesn't work for you – as long as you're giving your body a longer period of time to rest without food, you can still reap the benefits. You could start with 14/10 if that suits your life better.

*Dietary Intake Regulates the Circulating Inflammatory Monocyte Pool, August 2019

BLOOD SUGAR DIET

The blood sugar diet is another diet that has been hitting the headlines, with reported benefits of weight loss and improved blood sugar levels. High blood sugar levels can increase inflammation in the body and contribute to chronic illness. Therefore, the general principle of the blood sugar diet is likely to help with your anti-inflammatory lifestyle.

It is quite similar to the Mediterranean diet, following the principles of a high intake of fruits, vegetables, oils and nuts, while removing processed, fatty and unhealthy foods. It is quite a low-carb diet, which it describes as being more beneficial for your health than a low-fat diet.

What does differ from the guidance we've outlined in this book is the focus on weight loss. The literature suggests that to improve your blood sugar levels, it's important to reduce excess fat, which it says can clog up your liver and stop it working effectively. It suggests that if you have a lot of weight to lose, the starting diet is around 800 calories a day to drain fat from your organs, either every day or in a 5:2 fast. It also supports an increased level of exercise.

This type of extremely low-calorie diet is aimed at those who have a lot of weight to lose, but cutting calories dramatically can make it hard to sustain and increase cravings. It's best to get advice from your doctor before embarking on extreme calorie reduction.

If your goal is to reduce inflammation, then it's better to focus on removing ultra processed and inflammatory foods from your diet, and increasing the amount of anti-inflammatory foods you eat. You might find that eating in this healthful way promotes weight loss, if that is right for you, in a gentle and sustainable way.

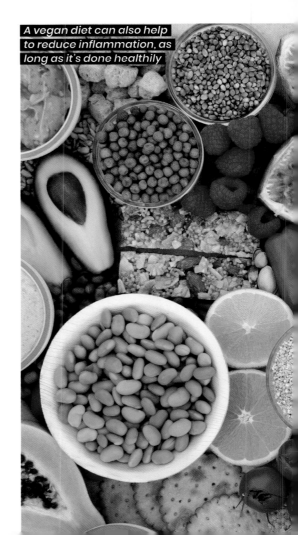
A vegan diet can also help to reduce inflammation, as long as it's done healthily

Don't forget to think about what you drink – both water and herbal teas are great on all these diets.

You may be thinking about moving to a more plant-based lifestyle – this can also help with inflammation. Both vegan and vegetarian diets will eliminate meat and fish, so you are already cutting out a big chunk of inflammation-causing foods (for example, processed meats). A vegan diet will also eliminate all other animal products, including dairy, eggs and honey. Some studies have shown that following a vegan or vegetarian diet can lead to lower levels of inflammation in the body.

However, it's not as simple as just removing animal products from your diet. It's possible to be plant based and still eat a lot of inflammatory foods. This is in part due to the huge rise in vegan alternatives on the shelves, such as 'fake meat' products. Many junk products are already vegan by their nature, including some crisps and biscuits. Therefore, if you opt to follow a vegan or vegetarian diet, and want to reduce your inflammatory response, then you'll still need to follow the basic rules in this book.

Rather than replacing your meat for processed meat substitutes, try to increase your intake of minimally processed soy, like tofu or tempeh, beans, lentils and grains. Base your meals around plants as far as possible, filling your plate with fruits and veg. You will still need to make an effort to introduce anti-inflammatory foods, such as healthy oils and fats.

There is a misconception that it can be expensive to follow a plant-based diet, but at its core, it's actually quite affordable. You don't need pricey protein powders or supplements, high-end grains or premium fruits. You can eat a healthy plant-based diet with everyday ingredients. Look out for fresh fruits and vegetables on offer and bulk buy complex carbohydrates. You can batch cook simple plant-based meals at home and they will last a long time too.

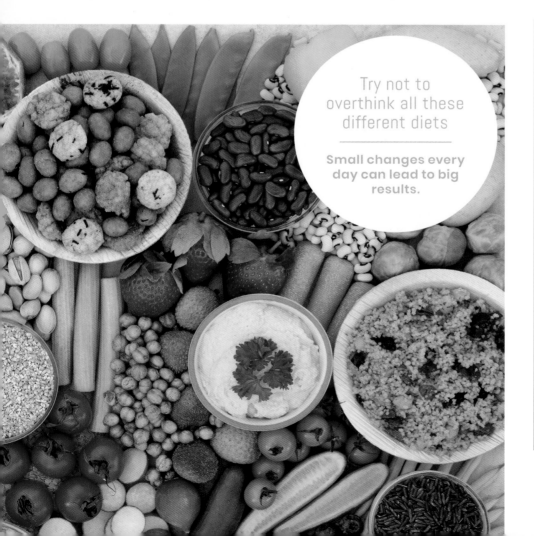

Try not to overthink all these different diets

Small changes every day can lead to big results.

The final word

There are many diets out there that can help you to take control of inflammation, but many are complicated and hard to follow, and you're more likely to fail if there are too many rules. At their core, a lot of these diets are promoting the same things – good, healthy, balanced foods. Saying that, if you do want to follow a diet to help you get to grips with eating in a new way, some of these diets mentioned can ease you into your new lifestyle and provide tips and recipes along the way. You may also find online communities for these specific diets where you can meet like-minded people, share advice and get support from others.

© Getty

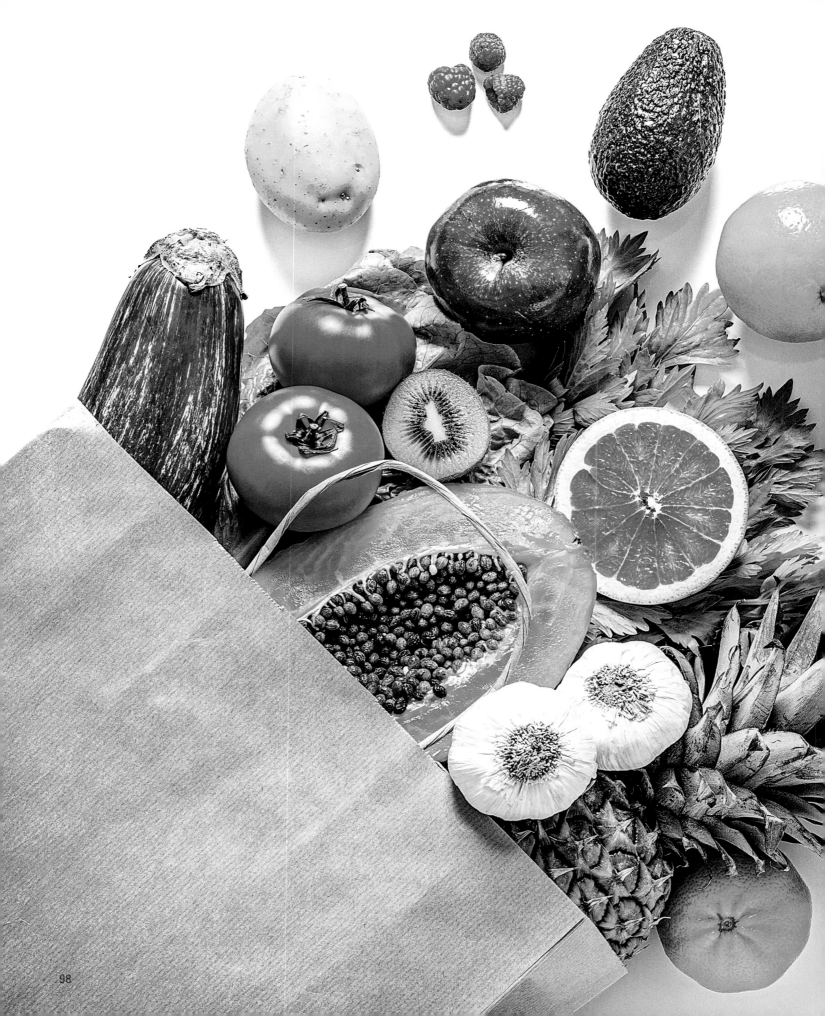

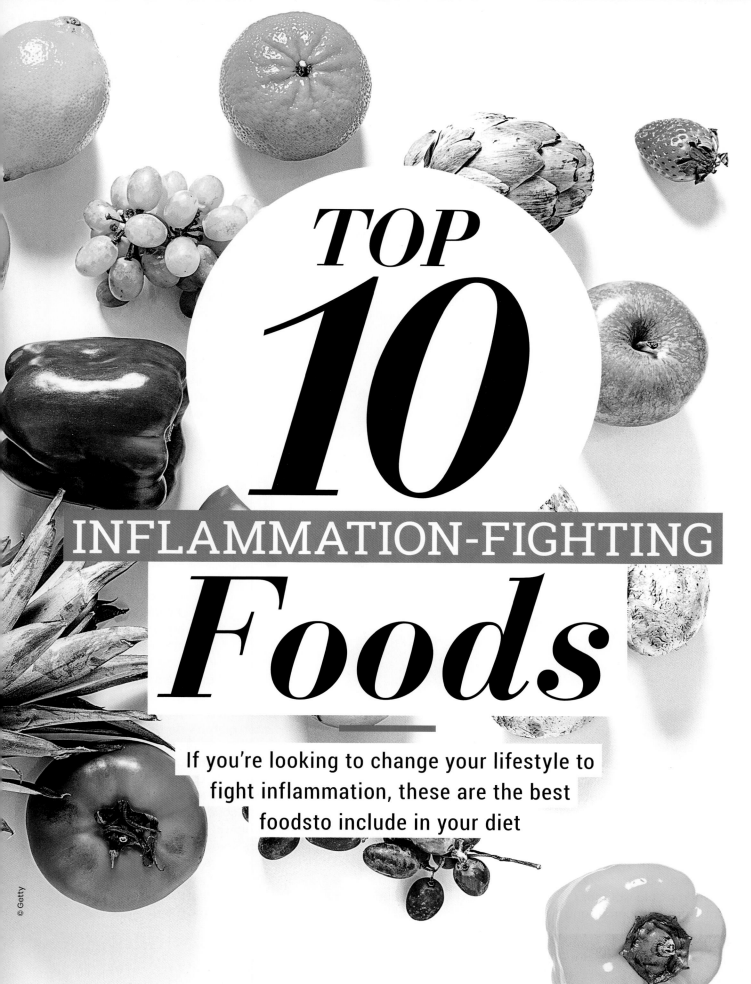

TOP
10
INFLAMMATION-FIGHTING
Foods

If you're looking to change your lifestyle to fight inflammation, these are the best foodsto include in your diet

© Getty

99

One of the best foods to include in an anti-inflammatory diet is fruit. It's versatile, accessible and can also be quite cheap – you can even try growing your own. It's best to try to eat a variety of fruits every week, aiming to consume as many different colours as possible. The more colours you can eat, the more nutrients, vitamins and antioxidants you're getting in your body – all of which will help with inflammation.

It's a good idea to eat with the seasons if you can. Fruits that are naturally in season will tend to be the most nutrient dense as they thrive in certain conditions and at certain times of the year. This also helps you to get a good enough variety, as seasonal fruit changes throughout the year. Try shopping at your local greengrocer or farmers' market if you can, as you'll get more of a sense of what's in season when, rather than the supermarket, which imports fruits all year round.

While all fruits can help in the fight against inflammation, some have even more benefits than others. Berries are top of the anti-inflammation list, as these are crammed with antioxidants and vitamins. They are also good for boosting your fibre intake, which we know is beneficial from an anti-inflammation and disease-prevention point of view. Any berry is a good choice, including strawberries, blackberries, raspberries, cranberries and blueberries. You could even try picking your own when they're in season, or foraging in the countryside. They are great as a snack to eat just as they are, or you could have them as a pudding mixed with a little yogurt and honey or with your breakfast. Frozen berries are handy for adding to smoothies or porridge too, so keep a couple of mixed bags in your freezer.

Citrus fruits are also a good

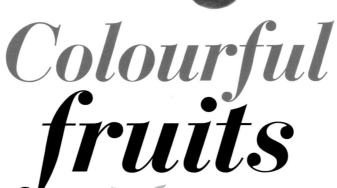

Colourful fruits

option, helping to boost your vitamin C intake, as well as other anti-inflammatory nutrients. Try adding in grapefruit or orange, lemons or limes. You might like to add slices to a glass of water to give your drink a fruity kick. Grapefruit can make a good breakfast option, and oranges are a handy snack.

If you're looking to get plenty of fibre in your diet, try to eat bananas, apples and pears – these are all full of fibre, as well as other nutrients. Apples and pears are great as a sweet pudding option, baked and served with a yogurt and some raisins. Bananas are a perfect pre-exercise fuelling option, as they are carb heavy – sliced banana and nut butter on some wholegrain bread offers a great blend of carbs, fats and protein. You can also mix in some stone fruits, like peaches, apricots, plums or cherries, which have all been linked to having anti-inflammatory benefits.

All fruit is going to be beneficial for your diet when looking to reduce inflammation, so choose fruits that you enjoy, and maybe set yourself a challenge to try a new fruit every month. Fresh is best if you can, but don't be afraid to use frozen fruit either, which can sometimes work out cheaper. Frozen fruit is often picked when it's at its peak, so the nutrients are locked in.

Dried fruits can be handy as a snack option and are good for adding fibre, but the sugar is quite concentrated and they can be high in calories for how much they fill you up, so eat them more sparingly. A portion is around 30g, and it's worth learning what that looks like so you don't overconsume them.

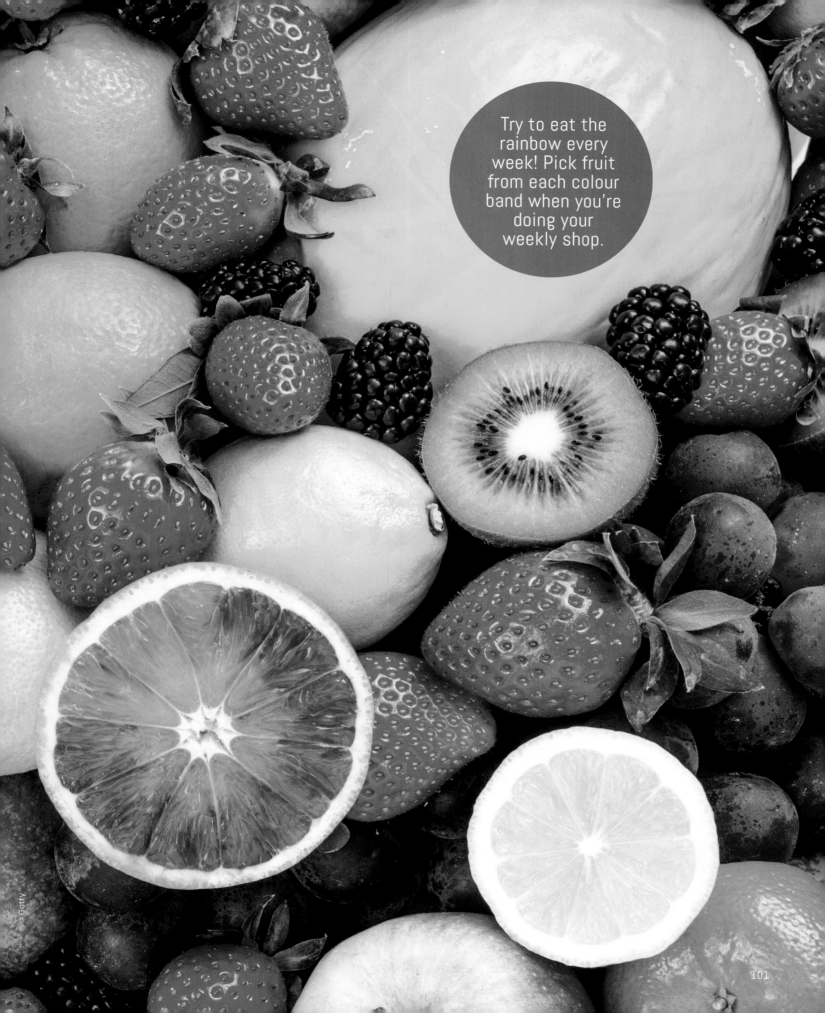

Try to eat the rainbow every week! Pick fruit from each colour band when you're doing your weekly shop.

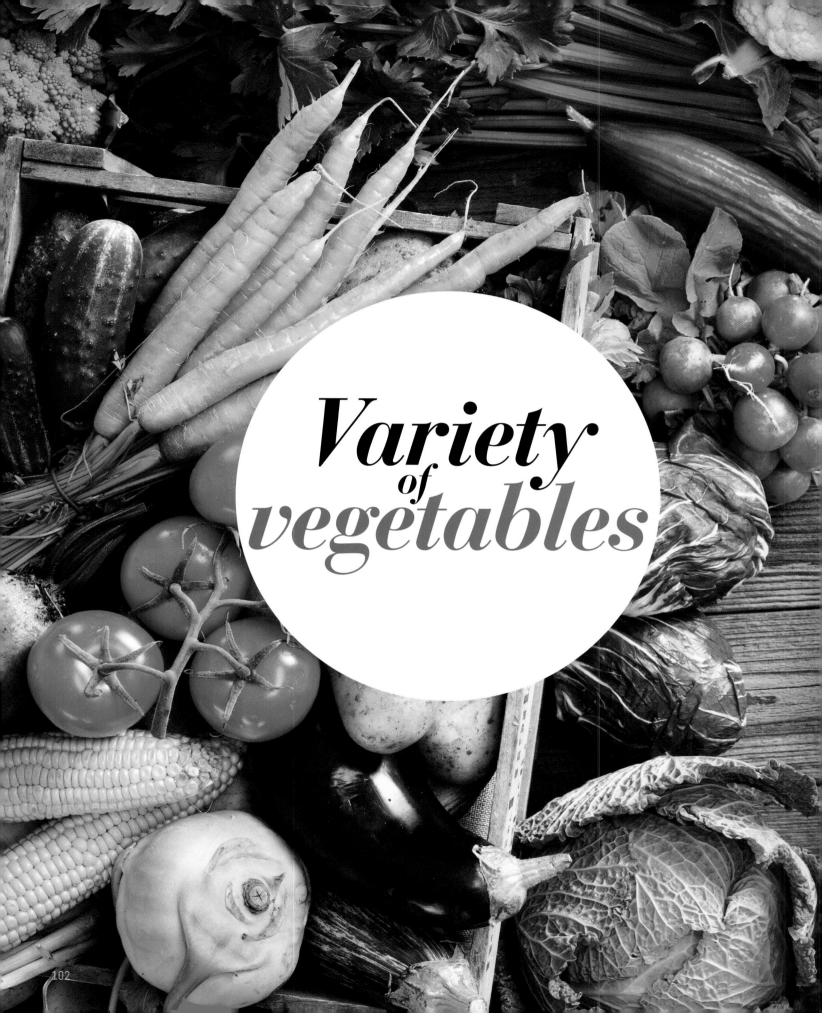

Variety of *vegetables*

Just like fruit, vegetables are a key component of an anti-inflammatory diet, and again the important thing is to try to eat a wide variety.

Vegetables fall into two main types – starchy and non-starchy – and both play a part in an anti-inflammatory diet. Starch is a carbohydrate – the main one that we have in our diets. You might have also heard of the term 'complex carbohydrate' – this refers to carbohydrates that contain long chains of sugar molecules that take longer to break down and digest than simple carbohydrates. Complex carbohydrates help you to feel more energetic for longer, as well as fuller for longer. Starch is one of these complex carbohydrates. Ideally, we want to eat a mix of both starchy and non-starchy veg to get the best mix of nutrients and vitamins.

Starchy vegetables that you should try to include in your diet include things like potatoes, sweet potatoes, all kinds of squash and pumpkin, parsnips, peas and corn. All of these vegetables are packed with antioxidants and also many important vitamins and minerals, including potassium and vitamin K. This means that they contribute to an anti-inflammatory response in the body, as well as helping to increase your fibre intake. Starchy forms of vegetables tend to be higher in calories per portion, so they need to be incorporated into a balanced, healthy diet. Starchy vegetables are good as a base for a meal. If you need a quick and easy dinner, you could try something like a baked sweet potato, topped with mixed beans and hummus. Starchy vegetables also make a great base for a soup, meaning you can get lots of different varieties in one easy meal.

The other type of vegetable is non-starchy. These are high in nutrients and low in calories, so you can fill your plate with them. In this category you will find things like broccoli, salad vegetables, spinach, peppers, onions, mushrooms and so on. These types of vegetables also have a high water content, so are great for keeping your body hydrated. They still have a good amount of nutrients, vitamins, minerals and antioxidants. They are low in carbohydrates and so they have little impact on your blood sugar levels.

When picking your non-starchy vegetables, they are all beneficial, but some have even better anti-inflammatory properties. For example, broccoli is shown to be rich in an antioxidant called sulforaphane, which helps to decrease inflammation. Bell peppers of all colours have another antioxidant called quercetin, which is again associated with a lower level of inflammation and disease prevention. This is why

> 66
> ## Add vegetables into smoothies to boost your nutrient intake on the go

it's so important to eat a good mixture of vegetables – they all have slightly different types of nutrients, so a variety means you get all of them in your body to maximise the benefits.

Fresh vegetables are best, but you can also get plenty of goodness from frozen options. It can work out cheaper to have some frozen vegetables in your freezer that you can dip into to complement your fresh vegetables and help you eat a bigger selection. You can also have some canned vegetables, like sweetcorn, and they are handy to keep in your cupboard for a quick vegetable option.

How you cook your vegetables is just as important. Deep frying your potatoes to make chips takes away from the health benefits and would undo the anti-inflammatory properties. It's better to bake, boil or steam your vegetables to keep as many nutrients in as possible. You can also eat many vegetables in their raw, natural state – think salad vegetables and crudités. We have a section in this bookazine that looks at different cooking methods in more detail in terms of anti-inflammatory benefits.

Try replacing pasta and noodles with veg-based options, like courgette sheets in lasagne or carrot noodles.

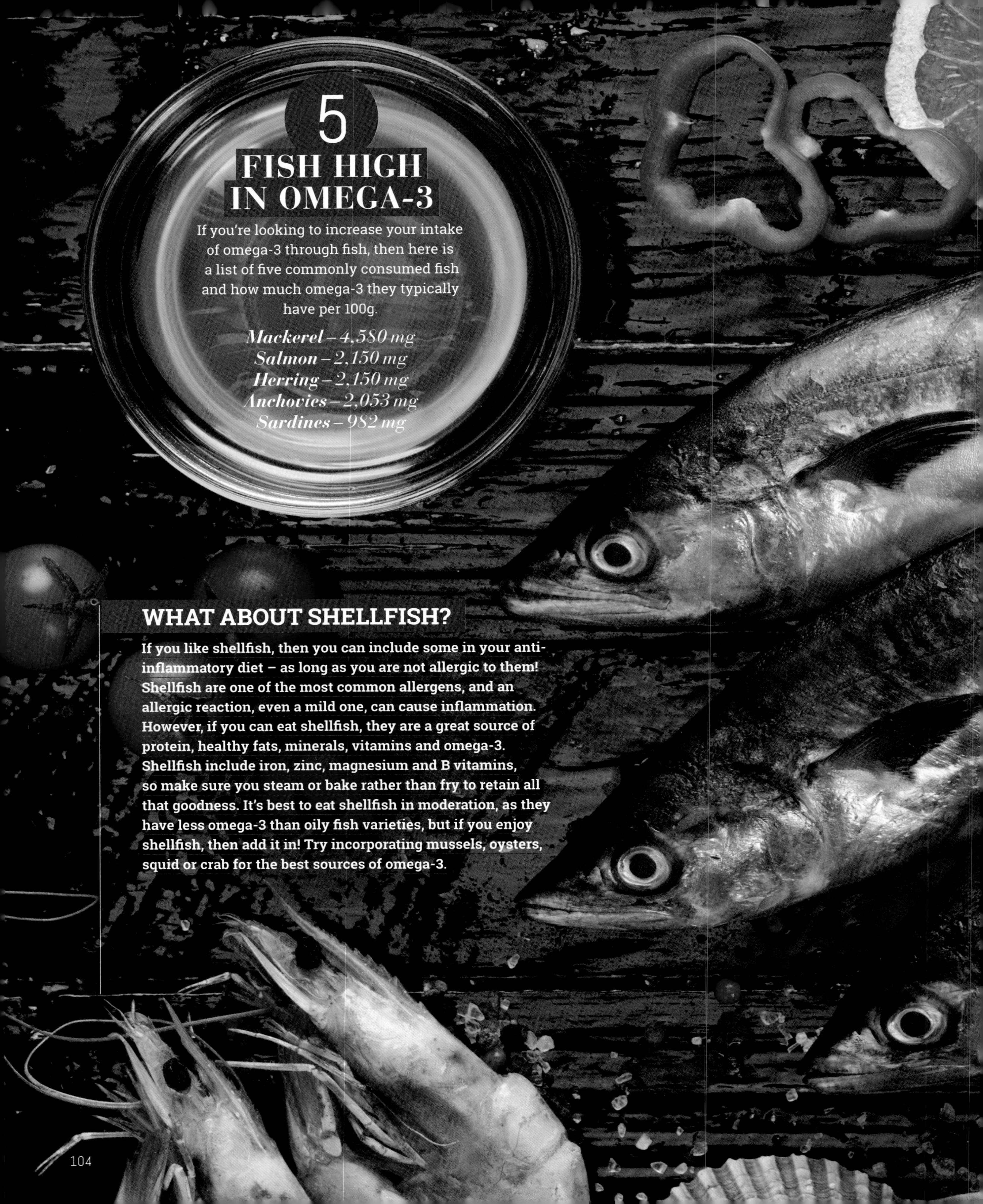

5
FISH HIGH IN OMEGA-3

If you're looking to increase your intake of omega-3 through fish, then here is a list of five commonly consumed fish and how much omega-3 they typically have per 100g.

Mackerel – 4,580 mg
Salmon – 2,150 mg
Herring – 2,150 mg
Anchovies – 2,053 mg
Sardines – 982 mg

WHAT ABOUT SHELLFISH?

If you like shellfish, then you can include some in your anti-inflammatory diet – as long as you are not allergic to them! Shellfish are one of the most common allergens, and an allergic reaction, even a mild one, can cause inflammation. However, if you can eat shellfish, they are a great source of protein, healthy fats, minerals, vitamins and omega-3. Shellfish include iron, zinc, magnesium and B vitamins, so make sure you steam or bake rather than fry to retain all that goodness. It's best to eat shellfish in moderation, as they have less omega-3 than oily fish varieties, but if you enjoy shellfish, then add it in! Try incorporating mussels, oysters, squid or crab for the best sources of omega-3.

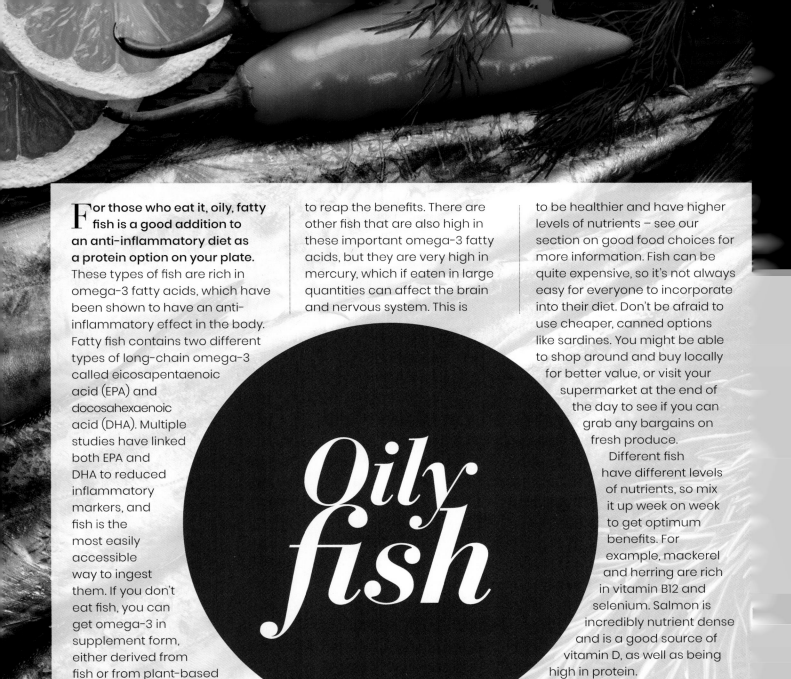

Oily fish

For those who eat it, oily, fatty fish is a good addition to an anti-inflammatory diet as a protein option on your plate. These types of fish are rich in omega-3 fatty acids, which have been shown to have an anti-inflammatory effect in the body. Fatty fish contains two different types of long-chain omega-3 called eicosapentaenoic acid (EPA) and docosahexaenoic acid (DHA). Multiple studies have linked both EPA and DHA to reduced inflammatory markers, and fish is the most easily accessible way to ingest them. If you don't eat fish, you can get omega-3 in supplement form, either derived from fish or from plant-based sources.

The best fish to eat are salmon, sardines, herring and mackerel, as these are rich in the omega-3 fatty acids we want to eat. Other fish to include are trout, sardines and anchovies. Try to eat around two portions of these kinds of fish every week to reap the benefits. There are other fish that are also high in these important omega-3 fatty acids, but they are very high in mercury, which if eaten in large quantities can affect the brain and nervous system. This is why it's recommended to stick to the smaller fish mentioned here, rather than larger fish, like swordfish or shark.

It is best to eat wild-caught fish where possible, as wild fish tend to be healthier and have higher levels of nutrients – see our section on good food choices for more information. Fish can be quite expensive, so it's not always easy for everyone to incorporate into their diet. Don't be afraid to use cheaper, canned options like sardines. You might be able to shop around and buy locally for better value, or visit your supermarket at the end of the day to see if you can grab any bargains on fresh produce.

Different fish have different levels of nutrients, so mix it up week on week to get optimum benefits. For example, mackerel and herring are rich in vitamin B12 and selenium. Salmon is incredibly nutrient dense and is a good source of vitamin D, as well as being high in protein.

Steam, bake or grill your fish to retain as many nutrients as possible – sadly, battered fish and chips isn't the most healthful option! Baked fish with steamed vegetables is a perfect, filling anti-inflammatory meal. One serving of fish is around 140g when cooked.

NUTRIENT-RICH WHOLEGRAINS TO TRY

If you want to optimise your diet and increase the anti-inflammatory effects of wholegrains, try incorporating different types of grain into your diet. Here are some alternative grains you may not have tried before – many of them are naturally gluten free. However, these are beneficial for anyone to eat. Many of these grains are quite cheap to buy in bulk, and can act as a filling base for your meals.

Buckwheat

A high-protein, gluten-free grain-like seed. Despite its name, it's not actually a grain at all, but you can cook with it in a similar way. You can cook it as a substitute for rice, but you can also find buckwheat flour, which can be used for all kinds of baking. It is rich in antioxidants, high in fibre and good for blood-sugar management.

Rye

Most commonly a type of bread, rye is richly flavoured, and it is related to wheat and barley (so it's not gluten-free, but it is low in gluten). Rye is rarely used as a grain on its own, due to its slightly bitter flavour. It can be used as a wholegrain (dark rye), or as a slightly refined version (light rye) to make different types of cracker, flatbread and bread.

Barley

There are two types of barley: pot barley and pearl barely. You will probably find it easier to find pearl barley, which has the husks removed and is easier to cook. You can use barley to make risotto as a rice substitute, and it is very nutritious. It's also quite cheap to buy and full of fibre. Pot barley is less common and harder to cook with its outer husk intact, but it does retain more nutrients and has a slightly nuttier taste.

Amaranth

Another pseudo grain, as such amaranth isgluten free. It is high in protein, which makes it a good option for those who are on a plant-based diet. It is an ancient crop and was loved by the Aztecs and Incas! It has a kind of malty aroma and nutty taste, and it can be hard to cook with. It can go quite 'gluey' when cooked, so it's often used to make a nutrient-rich porridge.

Millet

Another gluten-free grain option that comes in a few different varieties. Millet is thought to sustain around a third of the world's population, though it's not eaten as widely in the West. It can be used as an alternative to rice, but can also be used to make cakes, added to stews, or popped like popcorn for a snack.

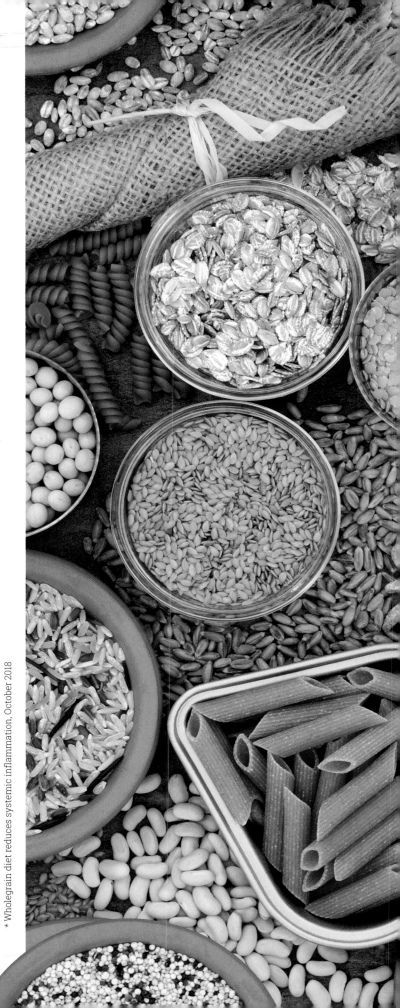

* Wholegrain diet reduces systemic inflammation, October 2018

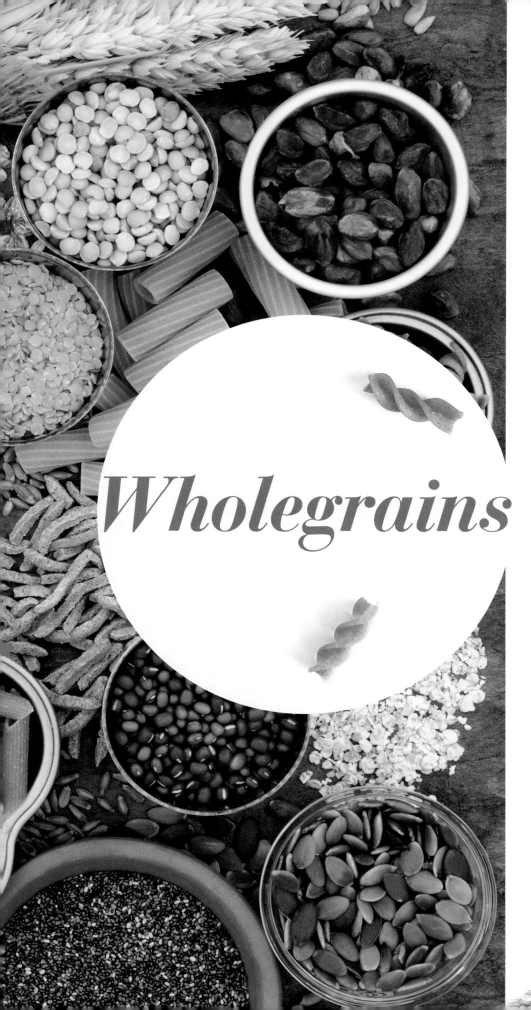

Wholegrains

An anti-inflammation diet is rich in wholegrains – that is grains that are wholly intact. A complete grain has three separate elements: the bran, which is the outer layer, rich in fibre; the germ, which is the inner part and is full of nutrients; and the endosperm, which is the central starchy part.

When these grains are heavily processed and refined, the bran and the germ are often removed, which leaves a simple, white grain. This is what is used for white flour, white bread and white rice, as well as in most processed foods. We know that eating ultra-processed foods increases inflammation in the body. However, eating wholegrain products can help to reduce inflammation, as wholegrains retain all the nutrients and goodness.

Wholegrains are rich in fibre, B vitamins, folic acid, protein, antioxidants and micronutrients. One meta-analysis* looked at nine different studies exploring a link between wholegrain consumption and a reduction in inflammatory markers. It concluded that, "The evidence suggested that citizens could benefit from increased whole grain intake for reducing systemic inflammation."

If you buy products that are listed as 'wholegrain', make sure you research what is actually in the product. Check the ingredients label to ensure the product uses the whole of the grain, and beware of terms like multigrain, which is a marketing term rather than a reflection of the product's contents.

© Getty

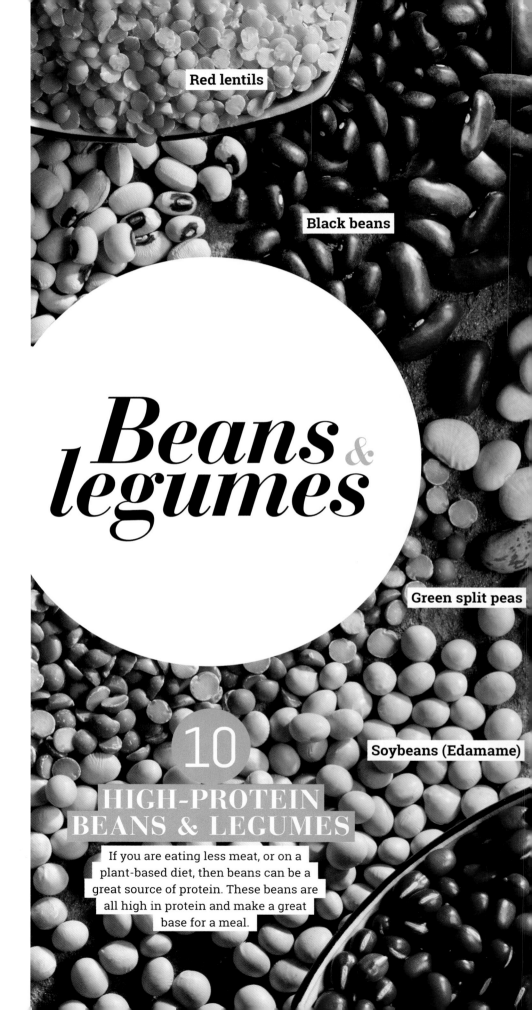

Red lentils

Black beans

Beans & legumes

Green split peas

10

HIGH-PROTEIN BEANS & LEGUMES

Soybeans (Edamame)

If you are eating less meat, or on a plant-based diet, then beans can be a great source of protein. These beans are all high in protein and make a great base for a meal.

Beans and legumes are a staple around the world, and it's no wonder! They are generally very cheap to buy, easy to cook with, and can be stored for a long time. Beans and legumes are a great source of protein, especially if you're on a plant-based diet, and they have a lot of fibre. They are also full of antioxidants, making them anti-inflammatory too. Beans have been shown to improve gut health, by increasing good bacteria levels. However, they can be hard to digest and some people might find it hard to break down beans in the gut, leading to gas and cramping. If this is the case, you may have to experiment; some people find lentils and peas easier to digest than beans.

Some people shy away from beans as they're not sure how to make them interesting, but there are so many things you can do with them beyond a mixed bean chilli (which is a great batch-cook option regardless!). Different beans, peas and legumes are at the heart of some great foods.

For example, falafel is made primarily with chickpeas (although you can use other types of beans too), as well as herbs and spices. Make sure you oven bake them rather than fry them to retain the health benefits. Serve them with some homemade houmous, again made from chickpeas, and you have a very bean-centric and tasty meal. Homemade bean burgers are very nutritious too, and can satisfy that craving for a burger! Lentils can be a pretty handy ingredient to learn to

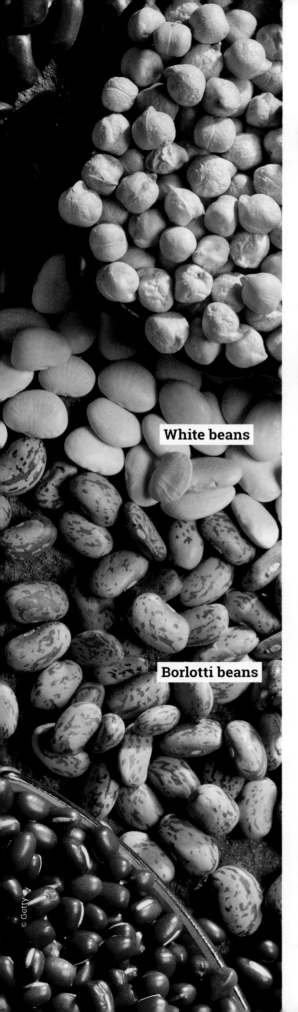

White beans

Borlotti beans

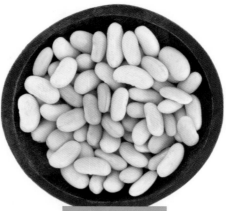

Haricot beans

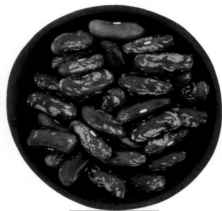

Pinto beans

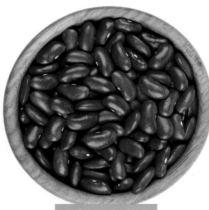

Kidney beans

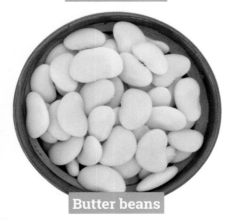

Butter beans

© Getty

cook with. They can be used to re-create some of your favourite dishes, such as lasagne or spaghetti Bolognese by creating a hearty Ragu that's meat free and rich in nutrients.

Beans can be used to make dips, like white bean dip, which usually bring in healthy fats like olive oil as well. You can also use beans as a base for a soup or a stew, which are perfect in the colder winter months to batch cook and freeze. Beans and legumes can be the star of the show in their own right, but they also make a great side dish for your protein. Beans and pulses also count towards one of your five a day (for one 80g portion – and you can only count one portion no matter how many you eat).

You can buy beans, peas and lentils as a dried option or canned. Dried varieties often need to be soaked before cooking, so they take a little longer to work with, but they are very cheap and can be stored for a long time. Canned options are ready to cook and so they can be used for a very quick and easy meal option.

You can also buy products that are made from beans. For example, tofu and tempeh, which are made from soybeans and act as a very nutritious and protein-rich alternative to meat. You can also get miso paste, which adds a rich umami flavour to foods and is made from fermented soy beans. If you're looking for a dairy-free alternative to milk, then soy milk made from soaking and grinding soy beans is a great option.

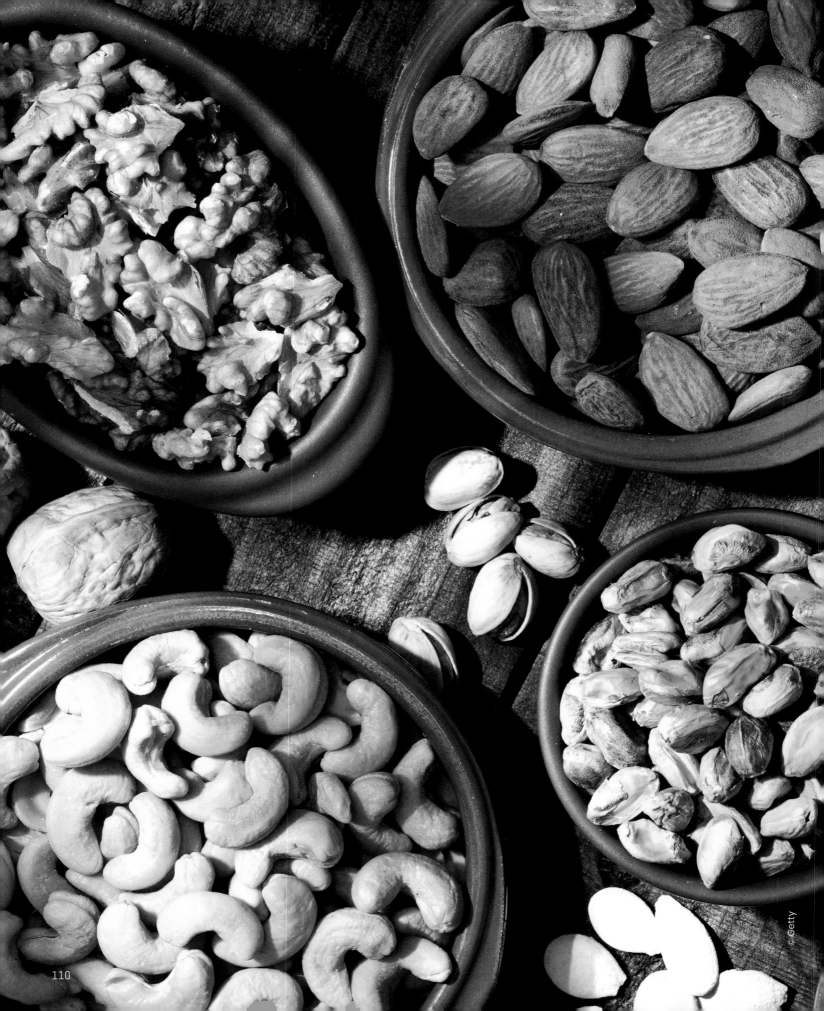

The simple nut is actually a really good anti-inflammatory food! Nuts are great as a snack, as they are easy to carry on the go, nutrient-dense, and offer a lot of energy in a small portion. They are high in calories, however, so you need to be careful how many you eat. Nuts are a source of healthy fats, which can help to lower cholesterol and reduce heart-disease risk, and they are anti-inflammatory. They are also a good source of protein, vitamins, minerals and antioxidants, as well as a source of omega-3 fatty acids. Depending on the nut variety, they are a great source of micronutrients too. Ideally, it's best to eat nuts in their most natural form – raw and unsalted. Aim for around 30g of nuts per day for optimum benefits, without too many calories.

There are so many nuts to choose from, so a variety is good to reap the benefits from each kind. Walnuts are one of the most nutritious varieties. For a start, they are high in ALA – alpha linoleic acid – a type of omega-3 fatty acid found in plant sources. It's thought that eating walnuts can lower the C-reactive protein (CRP), which is one of the key inflammatory markers and linked to things like arthritis and other inflammatory diseases. Walnuts are high in antioxidants and vitamin D, can support gut health and may help lower your blood pressure. All that from a nut!

Almonds are also a great nut to include in your diet, as they are high in fibre. This means that eating almonds can be a good option to help you feel full between meals, so they make

Nuts

Peanuts are technically a legume, the same as peas and beans but they are usually grouped with nuts.

a handy snack. They contain healthy fats, fibre, magnesium and vitamin E. If you're looking to reduce your dairy intake, almond milk is a good alternative for cooking, drinking and cereal.

Pistachios can be a bit of a pain to get out of the shell (although you can buy them pre-shelled, you often pay a lot more for the convenience), but it's worth persevering! They are popular in desserts and main meals, but great as a simple snack. They are also very nutritious, containing potassium, vitamin B6, healthy fats and protein. In fact, a serving of pistachios has the same potassium as half a banana. Pistachios contain a high level of antioxidants, meaning that they are very good for anti-inflammatory eating.

Brazil nuts are packed with antioxidants too, including vitamin E. They are also a good source of both calcium and magnesium for bone health, and selenium for brain health. They are high in calories, so eat them mindfully.

Nuts don't have to just be eaten as they are – there are lots of recipes that you can incorporate them into. For example, you could make granola bars with nuts as an on-the-go breakfast option. You can experiment with various nut roasts, for a plant-based alternative for your roast dinner. If you want to elevate your snacks, roast or gently toast nuts yourself in a mixture of spices. Nut butters are also a good option for a snack, on toast or to stir into your porridge. Just be careful when buying nut butters to make sure that they only contain the nuts themselves and not a lot of added ingredients.

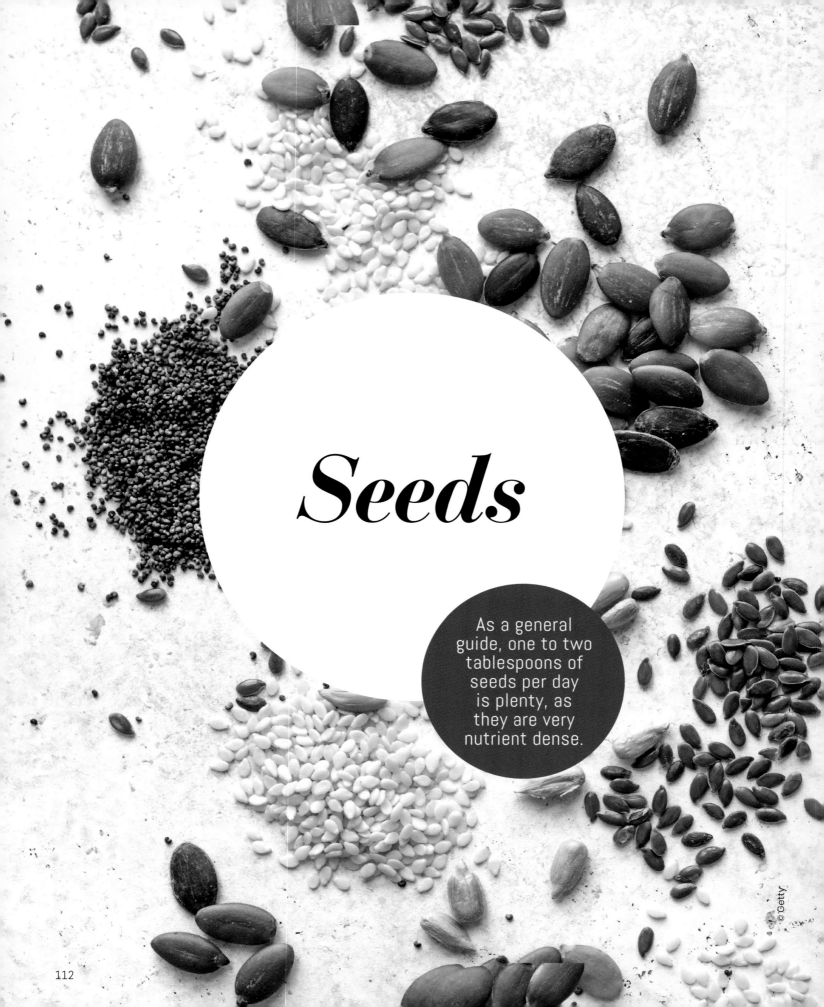

Seeds

As a general guide, one to two tablespoons of seeds per day is plenty, as they are very nutrient dense.

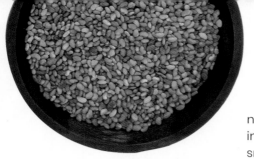

Seeds are incredibly nutritious, despite their small size. It's not surprising really – they have to contain all the nutritional information required to grow into plants! They are good for adding fibre into your diet, as well as healthy fats and micronutrients. You can have seeds as a snack, to create some great meals, or to sprinkle over your food for a crunchy topping. There are so many varieties out there, all with their own benefits, that any of them are worthy additions to your anti-inflammatory diet. You can even get some mixed seed packs so that you can enjoy multiple varieties simply and easily.

However, there are some seeds that do stand out as being particularly beneficial. Flaxseeds are one of the best to try and incorporate into your diet. This is because they are high in healthy omega-3 fats, which is great if you are plant-based and not eating fish. They are also high in fibre. Usually you buy flaxseeds ground or milled, rather than as whole seeds. This is because it is hard to digest the shell of whole flaxseeds and access those healthy fats. Flaxseed consumption has been linked to lower cholesterol levels, reduced blood pressure and lower blood-sugar levels. You can add milled flaxseed to porridge, a smoothie or over salads as an easy way to ingest it.

Another wonder seed is chia seeds. These seeds are also high in antioxidants and omega-3 fatty acids, making them naturally able to help reduce inflammation. Chia seeds are small, black seeds, but they swell up in liquid, which means that they can actually be quite filling. Due to their unusual texture in liquid, they are often used to make a 'chia pudding', which is a nutritious yet satisfying sweet treat – the chia seeds are added to any kind of milk and left overnight to swell up. You can add a sweetener like honey or agave syrup if you want to. You can then top with

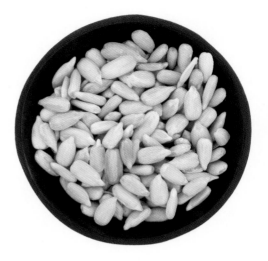

> ## "
> ## You can have seeds as a snack, to create some great meals, or to sprinkle over your food

fruit to serve the next day. It takes on an almost jelly-like consistency, and there are endless recipes out there to try different flavour combinations.

Pumpkin and sunflower seeds are both healthy options to add to your diet, too. Pumpkin seeds are popular, and for good reason. Not only are they tasty, but they have been linked to numerous health benefits, such as reducing blood pressure,

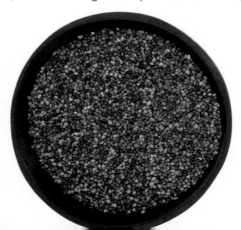

increasing good cholesterol levels, relieving menopausal symptoms and bladder health. Sunflower seeds are high in good healthy fats, vitamin E and protein, and have been associated with a reduction in inflammation in older people. You can eat both these types of seeds as a snack, but you can also bake with them in bread or cereal bars, for example. You can also opt to toss them in a little oil and some spices, then bake gently for a toasted snack. Even better, buy the pumpkin and use the flesh to make a soup, then scoop out the seeds, dry them out and gently roast them – it's cheaper than buying the packed versions in the shop!

Small seeds can be used to add flavour to your cooking. Nigella seeds are small, black seeds that add a lot of flavour to Indian and Middle Eastern recipes in particular. Or you can add sesame seeds on top of Chinese-based stir fries for a nutty crunch. Browse the herbs and spices aisle next time you're in the supermarket and you will find a whole host of seeds that can enhance your cooking, while adding in anti-inflammatory benefits.

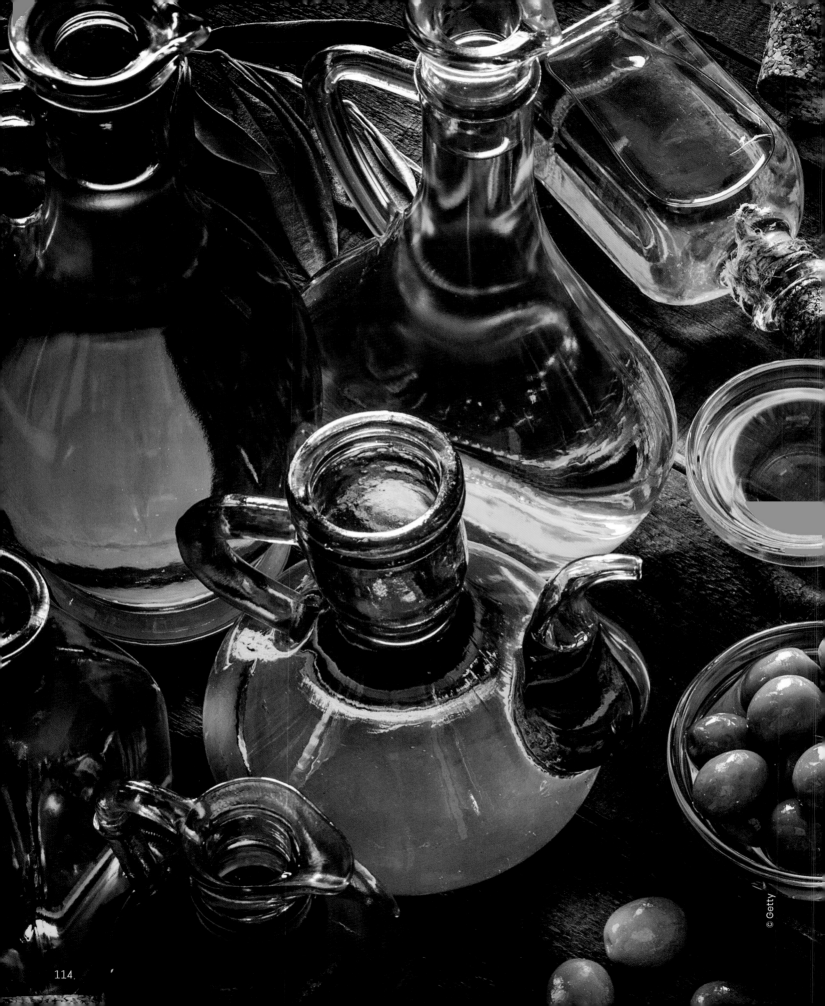

MAKE YOUR OWN INFUSED OILS

You can buy all manner of flavoured oils, but it's quite straightforward to infuse oil yourself. Flavoured oils are great for adding different flavours when cooking, but are best used as a drizzle over salads to retain all the flavours that might be lost when cooked. You can either make a cold infusion or a heated infusion.

Cold infusion

Simply add 1-2 tablespoons of dried herbs of your choice to oil, and mix together. It's best to prepare these in a glass jar with a lid. Store the oils in a cool, dark place to let them infuse, and attend every few days to shake the jar and check the strength of flavour. You will need to leave the jars for several weeks to get the intensity of flavour. Your herbs need to be fully dried using this method, so that there is no moisture for bacteria to breed.

Heated infusion

You can also make your infused oils a little quicker using the heated method. Heat the oil in a small saucepan to a medium heat. Add your chosen herbs or spices and allow to simmer gently for a few minutes. Turn off the heat and then pop a lid on, and leave to steep for a couple of hours. The longer it steeps, the stronger the flavour. Once you're happy with the strength of flavour, you can strain out the herbs or spices and pour into a glass jar for storage.

Healthy oils

If you're cooking your food in oil, then make sure that the oil is helping with your anti-inflammation diet too! Healthy fats are found in some oils; whereas other oils are highly processed and quite unhealthy. Knowing which oils to use can make a great difference to your cooking, as well as deliver enhanced health benefits.

Top of your list should be a very high-quality olive oil. Look for organic, extra virgin olive oil if you can, to get the most out of it. Olive oil is very rich in monounsaturated fats, specifically oleic acid, which has been linked to reduced inflammation. It is also packed with antioxidants, including vitamins K and E, which can help to fight inflammation and reduce your blood cholesterol. Olive oil is widely used in the Mediterranean diet, which is naturally anti-inflammatory due to its focus on healthy,

unprocessed foods. Olive oil can withstand quite high heats, so it is a good, stable oil to use for all kinds of cooking. However, it's also great as a cold oil and you can use it to drizzle over salads as a finishing oil. You can even use it in place of a butter or spread with bread, and mix with balsamic vinegar for a tasty dipping sauce.

While olive oil does get a lot of attention, there are other oils out there that are also good to cook with on an anti-inflammatory diet. Avocado oil is a great option, keeping many of the benefits that you can get from the avocado as a fruit with nutrient-rich healthy fats. Oils that are made from nuts and seeds are also a good choice, as these products are naturally high in healthy fats. Consider trying walnut oil, flaxseed oil or pumpkin seed oil, but you may see other options in the supermarket to try as well.

We have focused a lot on the things you can eat to reduce inflammation, but did you know that you can help to reduce inflammation by what you drink, too? Some teas can have a great effect on your body. They are a good way for you to stay hydrated as well as benefit from their nutritional properties.

The tea that is most often linked with anti-inflammation is green tea. Green tea is made from the leaves of the plant Camellia sinensis, which is the same plant that black tea comes from. Whereas black tea is made from fermented leaves, green tea is brewed from unprocessed and unfermented leaves, which give a bright-green colour from which the tea's name derives.

Green tea is popular in East Asia, where it is grown, and it dates back thousands of years as a drink with health benefits. The main reason that green tea is considered a health drink is due to compounds called polyphenols, which are present in tea. These polyphenols protect the body against diseases and are antioxidant. As green tea is unprocessed, it is higher in these plant compounds than other more processed teas. One of the most significant is called EGCG (catechins and epigallocatechin gallate), a flavonoid that is bioactive and very potent. Some studies have linked these compounds to boosting the metabolism and hence promoting fat burning, but this isn't the main focus of green tea's benefits. The polyphenols are also thought to help protect the brain from the effects of ageing, may reduce the risk of heart disease, may help manage cholesterol levels, and can control blood sugar levels. Green tea is caffeinated, though it contains a little less than black tea, so it's wise to drink it before midday so that it doesn't interfere with your sleep patterns.

Other teas have anti-inflammatory benefits, too. Even standard black tea has its place – it's thought that the fermentation process that turns the green leaves into black tea produces a different variety of flavonoids that can also help with inflammation, as well as lowering the risk of diabetes. If you prefer tea of a herbal variety, peppermint tea has no caffeine, and yet is packed with lots of flavonoids that can help to reduce inflammation. Peppermint tea is also good at aiding digestion, helping to maintain good gut health. If you have an upset stomach, or you feel unwell, ginger tea can help to soothe and reduce nausea and indigestion. It is also packed with antioxidants that could help reduce inflammation. And if you're looking for something to help you get off to sleep, look for a tea with chamomile, as this is caffeine free and has specific chemicals that reduce inflammation and relax the mind.

Tea

BREWING TEA CORRECTLY

In order to retain the health benefits of tea, you need to be careful when preparing it. Brewing your tea incorrectly can change the level of healthful compounds in your drink. Try to use fresh tea rather than tea bags, as this will have higher levels of antioxidants and also more flavour will come out when brewing. Black, dark oolong and herbal teas should be brewed

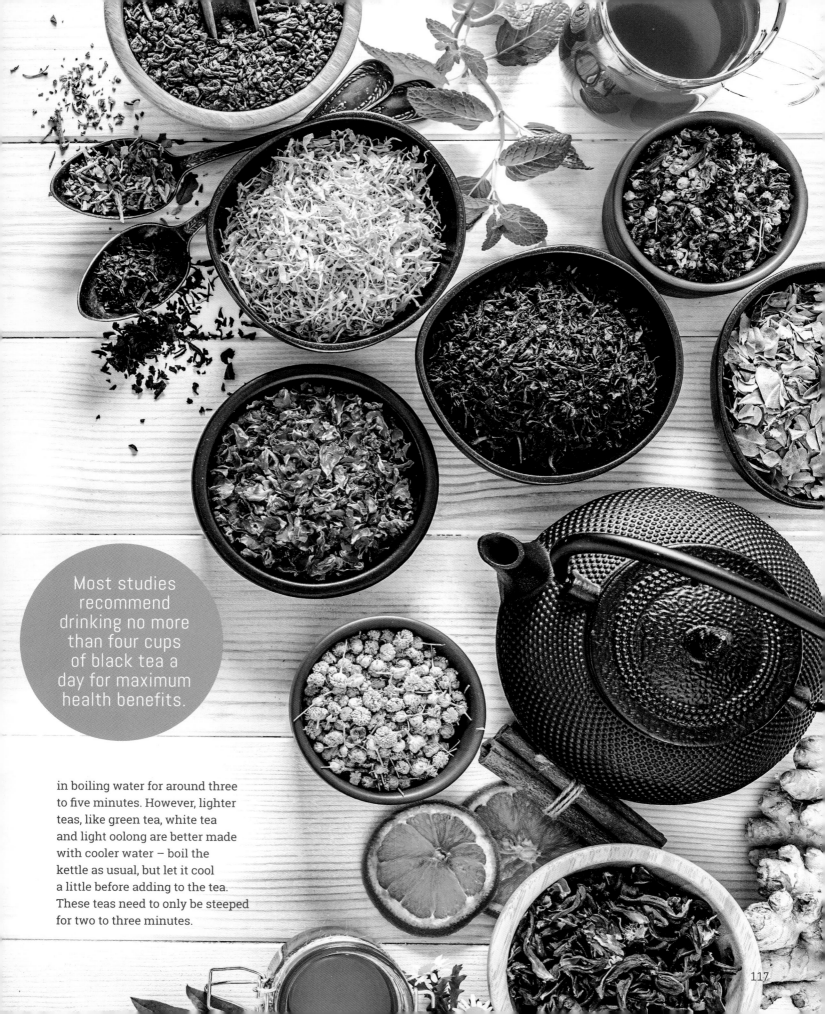

Most studies recommend drinking no more than four cups of black tea a day for maximum health benefits.

in boiling water for around three to five minutes. However, lighter teas, like green tea, white tea and light oolong are better made with cooler water – boil the kettle as usual, but let it cool a little before adding to the tea. These teas need to only be steeped for two to three minutes.

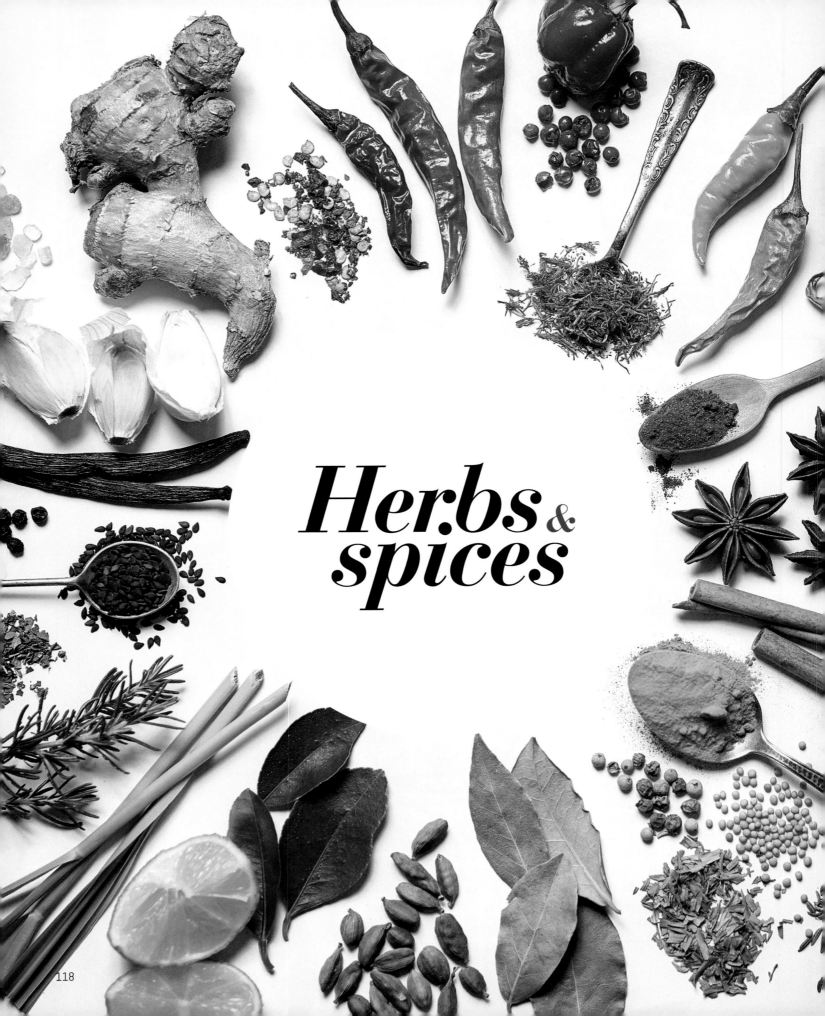

Herbs & spices

Store cupboard staples

Make sure that you have these herbs and spices to hand in your cupboard to easily add them to your meals when cooking and boost the anti-inflammatory benefits – and flavours – of your food:

Ground turmeric
Fresh root or dried ginger
Cinnamon powder
Fresh garlic bulbs
Black pepper
Cloves
Cardamon
Sea salt

Make your own anti-inflammatory spice blend by Mixing two or more complementary spices to use in your cooking.

Herbs and spices that you use for cooking can do much more than create great flavours! Many can actually reduce inflammatory markers in the body, so learning about the health benefits of these can help you to incorporate them into your meals. Herbs and spices are generally quite cheap to buy and can be used sparingly, so it's a cost-effective and accessible way to introduce anti-inflammatory compounds into your diet.

Turmeric is often touted as an anti-inflammatory, and is especially popular in Indian cuisine thanks to its rich flavour and deep colour. It has more than 300 active compounds in it, including the one that most people have heard of: curcumin. You can buy supplements with high amounts of curcumin, far more than you could get out of the spice itself. Most of these supplements will also contain black pepper, as this increases curcumin absorption. You can also include turmeric in your cooking – you might not get much curcumin from a teaspoon of the spice, but it's still beneficial and flavoursome, and you can benefit from all the other compounds too.

Ginger is another spice that is great to include in your cooking. You can buy it fresh, which is best if you can so as to retain as many nutrients as possible. You can also get it dried, frozen, minced or powdered. It is widely used in traditional medicine too, to relieve nausea. It has more than 100 active compounds in it, which may help to reduce inflammation in the body. You can get it in supplement form, but it's easy to add to meals. It's great in soups, stews, stir fries and curries.

The humble garlic clove is a staple of many recipes, adding flavour and taste to meals. It can also help the body to fight off colds, by boosting the immune system. The active compounds found in garlic may help to reduce blood pressure too, as well as improve cholesterol levels. Garlic has antioxidants, which can reduce inflammation, and contains vitamins B6 and C.

When it comes to herbs, rosemary is a great one to start with. Rosemary has long been known for its medicinal properties and is native to the Mediterranean, so is often used in food around that region. It is high in manganese, which can help the body heal from injuries quickly, and it also contains carnosic acid, which is a potent antioxidant. Rosemary can even boost your immune system, reduce stress and improve your memory and focus. It has quite a distinctive taste, and you can buy it fresh or dried. You can even grow it yourself, adding fragrance to your garden.

You won't eat enough of any of these spices to get huge benefits from just one serving, but by adding in lots of herbs and spices to your cooking on a regular basis, you can start to reap some of the rewards. Having a good supply of herbs and spices at home can also help you to enhance your meals, making you more likely to enjoy them and get the most out of the nutrients of the whole meal.

© Getty

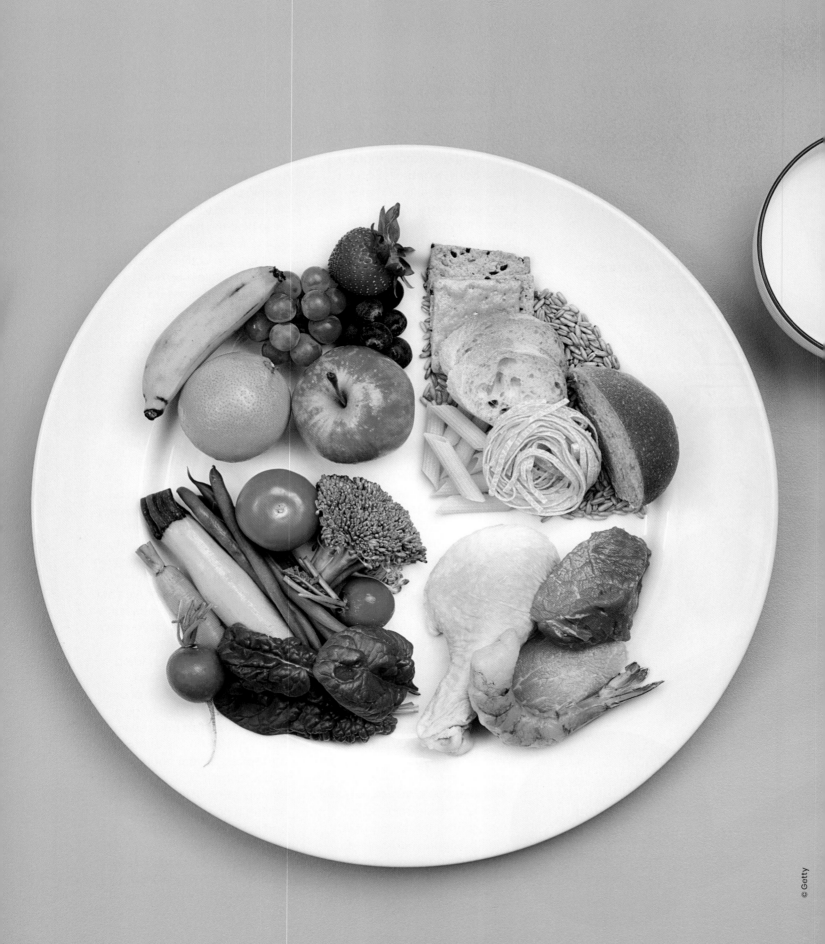

Key
ANTI-INFLAMMATORY
NUTRIENTS

The makeup of your food matters – we explore the key nutrients to help reduce inflammation

The anti-inflammation diet is based around healthy, nutrient-dense foods. Getting a balance of all the key nutrients is incredibly important in helping your body fight and reduce chronic inflammation.

There are two main types of nutrients in the food we eat: macronutrients and micronutrients. When you're aiming to eat in an anti-inflammatory way, you need to consider all of these. Macronutrients are broad categories, comprising the nutrients we need in large quantities for our health: fats, proteins and carbohydrates. This is the basis of all our meals. Micronutrients are only needed in small amounts, but are just as important. We usually get our macronutrients and micronutrients at the same time in a balanced diet.

Macronutrients for anti-inflammation

You may have heard of 'counting macros', which is a way of describing the amount of fats, proteins and carbohydrates you eat in a day. Usually this is based on a ratio, so 50/30/20 means you get 50% of your calorie intake from carbohydrate sources, 30% from protein and 20% from fat. This kind of precision isn't usually required unless you have a specific health or weight goal. For most people, it's important to ensure that you have a good amount of all the macronutrients from healthy sources. Each of the main macronutrients can help with inflammation.

You might have heard that carbs can trigger inflammation, but that's a broad statement that is somewhat inaccurate. It's true that some carbohydrates can contribute to higher levels of inflammation, but this is referring to refined carbohydrates. This means things like white bread and rice, pastries, biscuits, sugary drinks, sweets, chocolate, crisps, chips and so on. We already know that these highly processed foods are a big contributor towards inflammation in the body.

However, we need carbohydrates in our meals, as this is our body's primary source of energy. Complex carbohydrates (those that have not been heavily refined) help to reduce inflammation. This includes things like some vegetables, fruits, legumes, nuts, seeds and wholegrains.

These carbohydrates are a great source of dietary fibre. A high-fibre diet has been linked to lower levels of inflammation, and yet many of us don't eat enough in a day. An adult should aim for around 30 grams of fibre a day, but the average is around 18 grams. Fibre has been linked to a lower risk of heart disease, stroke, type 2 diabetes and bowel cancer. Fibre can also help our digestive system to work effectively, look after our gut health and make us feel fuller for longer. Try to have a high-fibre source of food at every meal, which can include things like porridge, wholegrain breads or pasta, pulses and legumes, vegetables and fruits with their skins on, and unsalted nuts. You

may want to use a food tracker app for a short period to log your daily meals and see what your fibre intake is like on a normal day to give you a starting point.

The next macronutrient to think about is protein. Protein is an essential part of our diet, helping to maintain, build and repair muscle. Again, protein can help you feel full, so you're less inclined to snack. You may need to track your protein, along with fibre, to make sure you're getting enough and make changes if you need to. Most adults need, on average, 0.75 grams of protein per kilo of body weight. You can get your protein from animal products or plant products to suit your dietary preferences. Think things like whole eggs, fish and lean meat, or beans, nuts and tofu.

Finally in the macronutrient category are fats. Ideally you want to get your fats from healthy sources that help to reduce inflammation in the body. There are good fats and bad fats – processed, long-life foods are going to fall into the latter category, and it's these types of fats that have a bad reputation. Don't be tempted to try a really low-fat diet, as you'll be missing out on the benefits of the good sources of fat. This includes extra-virgin olive oil, nuts, seeds, avocado and avocado oil, and oily fish.

There is plenty of overlap of foods in these categories, so you can plan a balanced meal quite easily that covers all these bases. However, different foods can vary a lot in the micronutrients that they offer, so let's look at these in more detail.

TAKING SUPPLEMENTS

You can get most of what you need through your food, but you may wish to try some supplements to help with inflammation if you're struggling to get on top of your diet, exercise, sleep and stress. Supplements aren't a miracle pill, but they might give you the additional support you need. There are quite a lot of supplements out there, and it can be hard to figure out which ones to try. If you don't get enough omega-3 from your diet, this is one area you could supplement in. If you eat animal products, then look for a good-quality fish oil supplement. You can also get omega-3 supplements from algae sources, perfect if you are vegetarian or vegan. Another supplement to consider is vitamin D. Many of us don't get enough of it naturally, so a supplement is often recommended anyway. You don't need a really high dose – 400-800 IU (10-20 micrograms) a day is plenty, but you shouldn't take more than 4,000 IU (100 micrograms) a day, as this can be harmful.

© Getty

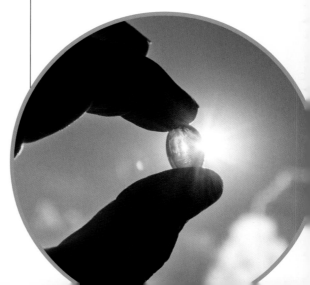

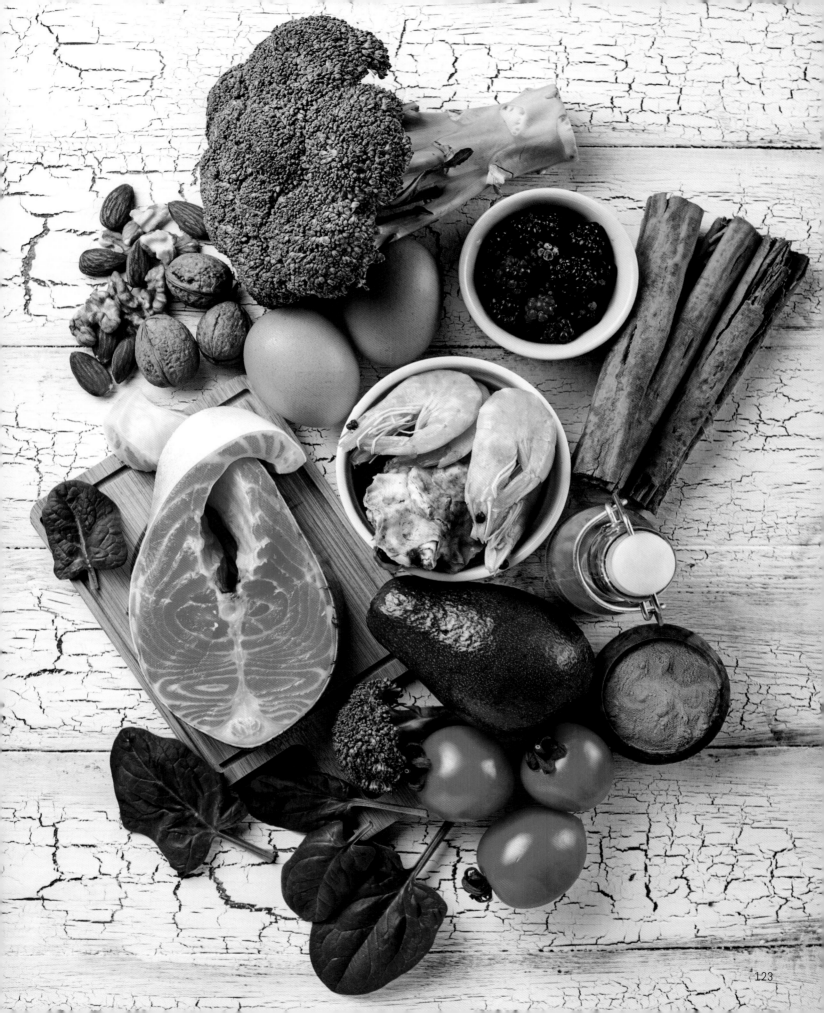

THE IMPORTANCE OF WATER

Water can often get overlooked, but when you're trying to reduce nflammation, it's actually very important. We need enough water to function. If we don't get enough, our body can start to struggle and this could even cause inflammation. There have been some studies to show that water can help to reduce chronic pain, which could be due to its anti-inflammatory effects. Staying well hydrated ensures all of your body's systems can work optimally, but adequate water intake also helps to flush out toxins and irritants that could otherwise cause inflammation. Plus, it's free! So it's win-win all round. Aim for eight glasses of water a day. If you do struggle to drink enough water, you could try infusing it with fruit to give it a subtle flavour, or try herbal teas instead. Don't be fooled by 'special' waters that claim to have certain health benefits – good old clean tap water is perfect.

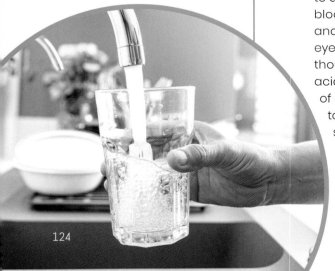

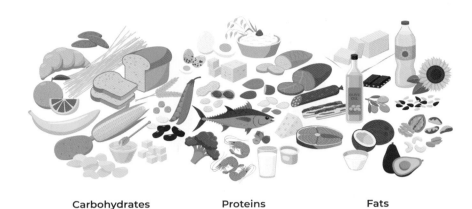

MACRONUTRIENTS

Carbohydrates   Proteins   Fats

A balance of the key macronutrients is important for reducing inflammation

Micronutrients for anti-inflammation

Micronutrients are the small nutrients that make up our foods. But just because they're small, doesn't mean they're not important. We need some key nutrients in an anti-inflammatory diet to get the best results.

Omega-3 is one of those key nutrients, which we know helps to reduce inflammation. In fact, omega-3 has been linked to a reduction in depression, blood pressure, heart disease and more. It can also improve eye health and brain health. It's thought that the omega-3 fatty acids reduce the production of certain molecules linked to inflammation. The best sources of omega-3 are oily fish like mackerel, salmon and herring. However, if you're plant based, you can also get omega-3 from flaxseeds, chia seeds, walnuts and soybeans.

Micronutrients include a range of vitamins and minerals. One of the micronutrients to consider is magnesium, which has a number of benefits, including a positive impact on your blood sugar levels. We have discussed elsewhere in this book how your blood sugar can impact on inflammation, so it's worth ensuring you do eat enough magnesium. Low magnesium intake has been linked to increased levels of inflammation, according to one report*. Good dietary sources of magnesium include green, leafy vegetables (e.g. spinach), legumes, nuts, seeds and wholegrains. Some foods, like cereal or bread, can be fortified with magnesium, but be careful

> Vitamin K could help to lower inflammation, so eat lots of leafy greens like kale and chard.

124

© Getty

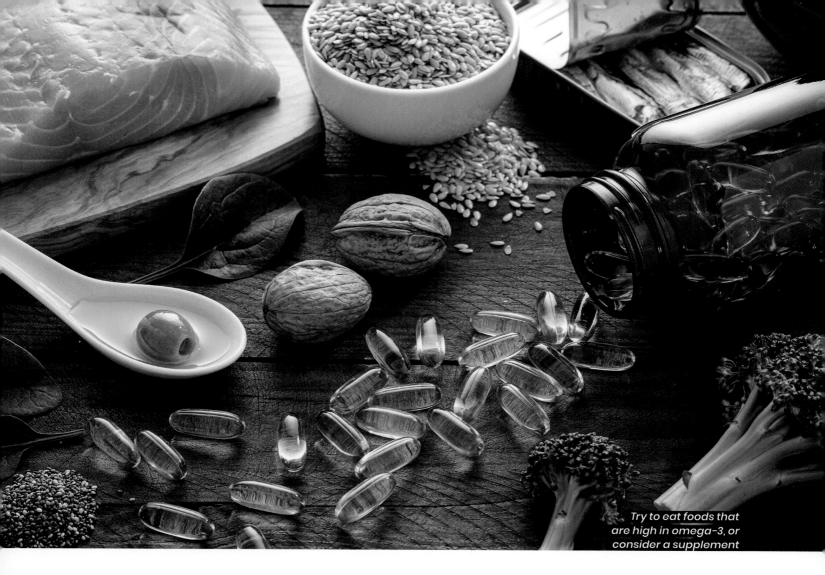

Try to eat foods that are high in omega-3, or consider a supplement

*Magnesium deficiency and increased inflammation: current perspectives, January 2018 **Vitamin D and inflammatory diseases, May 2014

with processed products as they may include many other inflammatory ingredients. You can get magnesium supplements, but it's quite abundant in plant foods.

When it comes to vitamins, you want a good mix for optimum health. Vitamin D has been shown in studies to be very important in the control of inflammation in our bodies**. Low levels of vitamin D have been linked to all kinds of diseases, such as inflammatory bowel disease and rheumatoid arthritis. However, it's hard to get enough vitamin D through diet alone. It is available in a few foods, like fatty fish, eggs and beef, as well as fortified foods like milk. Our primary source of vitamin D is via sunlight, so it's important to spend time outside to help your body produce enough. In parts of the world, we don't get enough sunlight, so a supplement is often recommended (see the information box on page 122).

B vitamins (like B6, B12 and B9 aka folate) are known as being good for your energy levels, but they could also reduce your levels of inflammation. You can get plenty of B vitamins in your normal diet, through things like fish, lean red meat, poultry, eggs and dairy products. If you are plant-based, then focus on fruits and vegetables, beans, peas and nuts. You shouldn't need to supplement if you eat a varied diet.

Vitamin E is an antioxidant and anti-inflammatory – found in sunflower seeds and almonds.

Vitamin C is an antioxidant, which means that it helps get rid of free radicals in your body. We know that antioxidants reduce inflammation too, so it's good to get plenty of vitamin C. This is easy if you eat a wide variety of fruits and vegetables. The best sources are citrus fruits, bell peppers, broccoli and leafy greens.

RECIPES

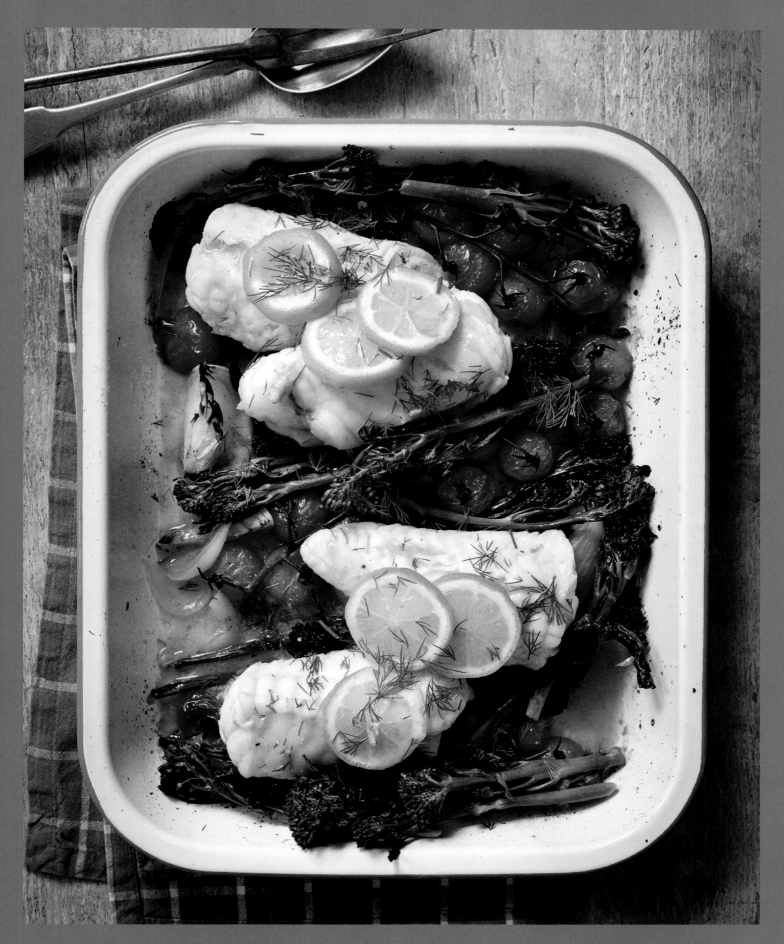

Lighter Thai green curry

This fragrant curry really packs a punch

Serves 4 • Ready in 30 mins

- 2tsp olive oil
- 200g baby aubergines, quartered
- 250g mixed veg (asparagus, baby corn, pak choi)
- 400ml can coconut milk
- 1-2tsp fish sauce
- juice of 1-2 limes

For the curry paste:

- 1 onion, roughly chopped
- 5cm piece ginger
- 3 garlic cloves
- 2 lemongrass sticks, roughly chopped
- 1 red and 1 green chilli, roughly chopped
- 1tsp ground coriander
- 2tsp fish sauce
- 2tsp palm sugar or honey
- large handful fresh coriander, including the stalks

To serve:

- sticky rice
- 2tbsp toasted coconut;
- 1 red chilli, sliced
- extra-fresh coriander leaves

1 Put 1tsp of the oil in a food processor with all the curry paste ingredients and whizz to a fine paste.

2 Heat the remaining oil in a wok and cook the paste until fragrant. Add the aubergines and coat, then cook for 3-4 mins until starting to soften. Add the remaining veg and cook for 2-3 mins.

3 Pour in the coconut milk and bring to the boil. Reduce the heat and simmer the sauce for 5-6 mins. Add the fish sauce and fresh lime juice to taste. Serve with sticky rice and topped with the toasted coconut, red chilli and coriander.

Per serving: 274 cals, 23g fat, 19g sat fat, 11g carbs

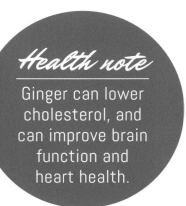

Health note

Ginger can lower cholesterol, and can improve brain function and heart health.

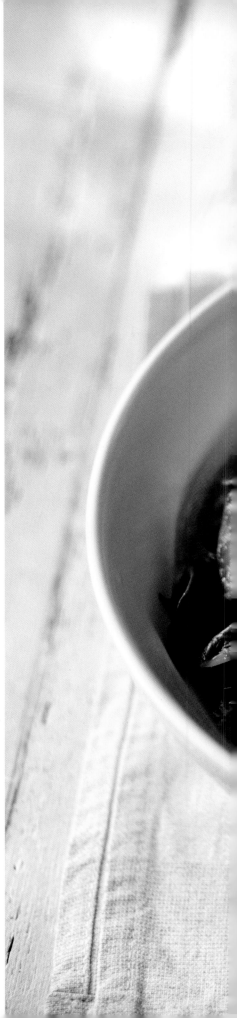

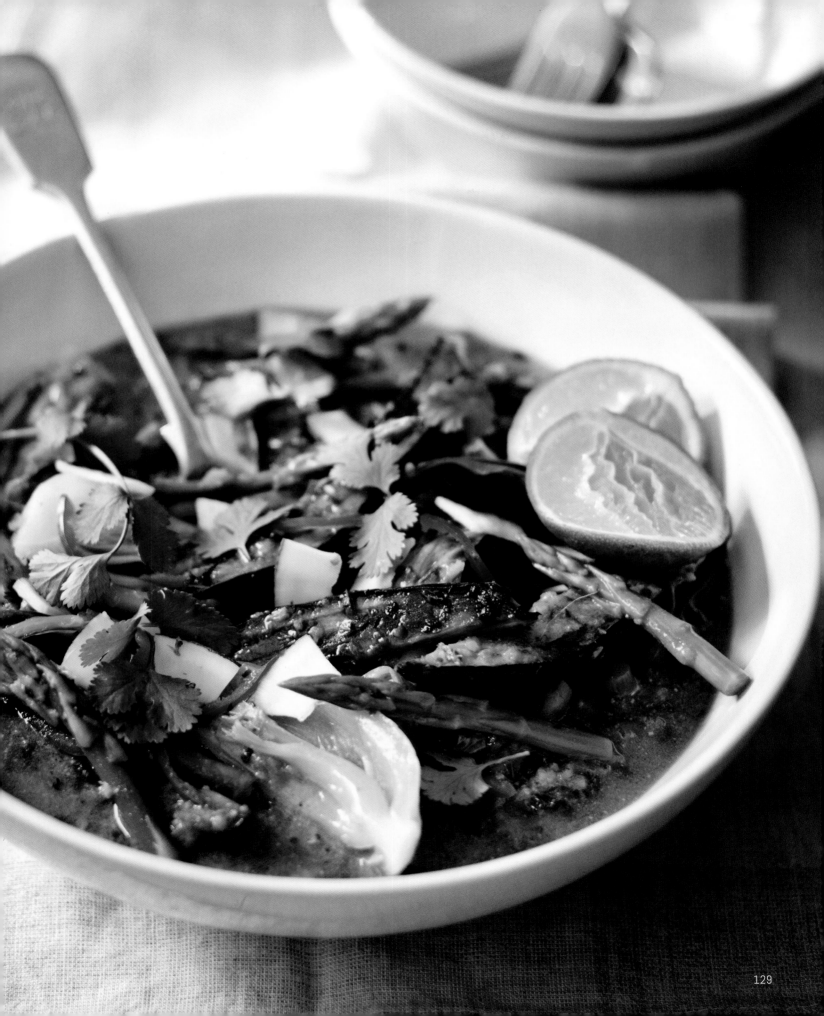

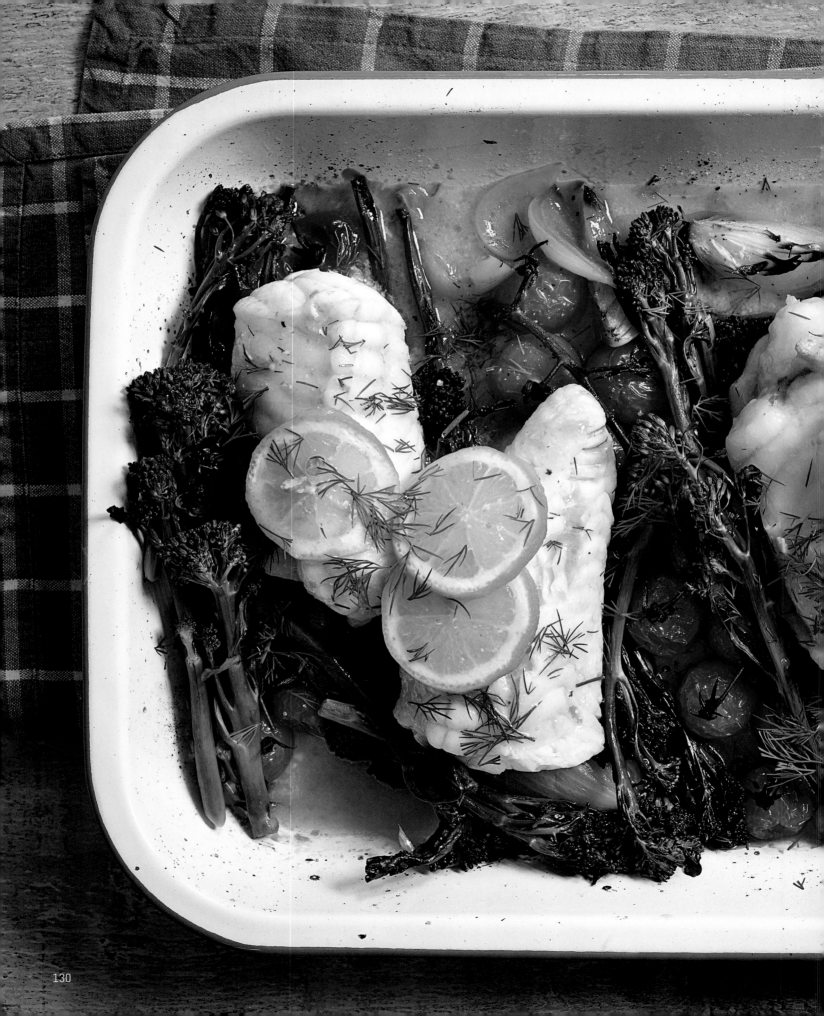

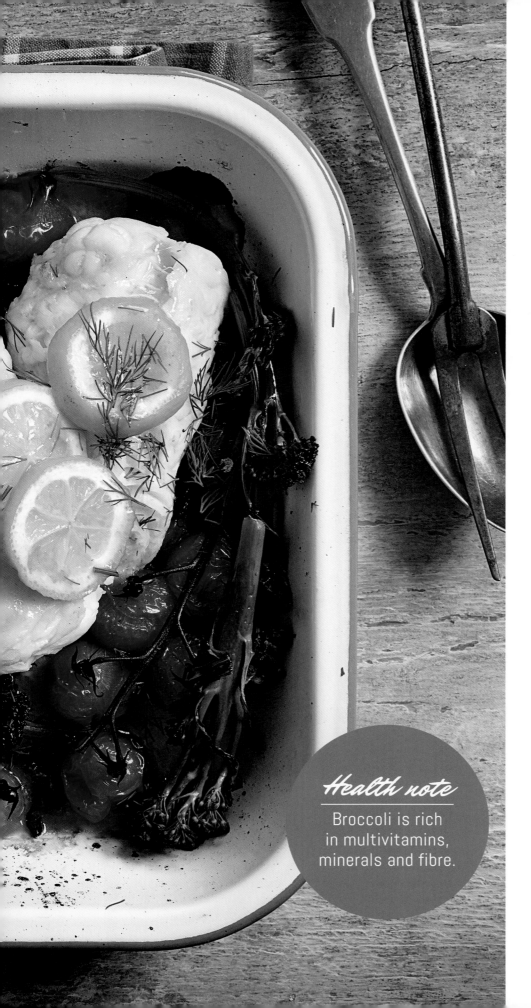

Fish and broccoli tray bake

Monkfish is full of flavour and texture, making it a perfect combination with the nutrient-rich vegetables in this dish

Serves 4 • Ready in 40 mins

- 1 onion, sliced into thin wedges
- 300g cherry tomatoes, on the vine
- 200g tenderstem broccoli
- 5tbsp good quality olive oil
- 4 x 150g pieces of monkfish fillet, chopped
- 1 lemon, sliced
- olive oil, for drizzling
- 1 small bunch of dill, roughly chopped

1 Heat the oven to 200C/Gas 6. On a large roasting tray, toss the onion, tomatoes and broccoli together with the olive oil. Bake for 20 mins until cooked through and slightly charred.

2 Place the fish on top of the veg and add the lemon slices and a little drizzle of oil.

3 Return to the oven for 15 mins until just cooked through. Remove and serve, topped with chopped dill.

Per serving: 292 cals, 15g fat, 2.5g sat fat, 7g carbs

Health note

Broccoli is rich in multivitamins, minerals and fibre.

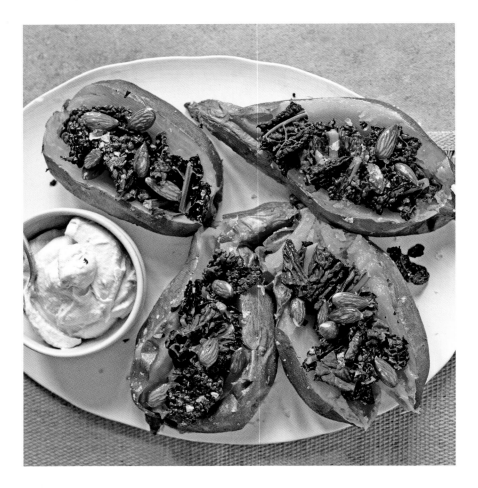

Lentil dal with charred courgettes

A comforting winter warmer

Serves 4 • Ready in 1 hr 15 mins

- 250g brown lentils, rinsed
- 1 litre vegetable stock
- 1 onion, thinly sliced
- 2tbsp olive oil
- 4 garlic cloves, crushed
- 4cm piece of root ginger, peeled and cut into matchsticks
- 1-2 green chillies, thinly sliced
- 60g tomato puree
- 3 courgettes, sliced
- 1tsp garam masala
- 160ml can of coconut cream a handful of coriander leaves, chopped
- steamed basmati rice, and coconut yogurt (optional), to serve

1 Bring the lentils and stock to the boil in a pan, cover and simmer for 1 hr. Fry the onion in 1tbsp oil over a medium-low heat for 6 mins, or until starting to brown.
2 Add the garlic, ginger and chillies, and cook for a further 2 mins.
3 Once the lentils have been cooking for 30 mins, add most of the onion mixture (reserving a little to garnish), the tomato puree and a good pinch of salt to the pan. Keep simmering for the next 20 mins of cooking time or until tender.
4 Heat the remaining oil and pan-fry the courgettes for 10 mins, turning until tender. Stir in the garam masala and coconut cream; cook for 10 more mins.
5 To serve, top the dal with the courgettes and a sprinkling of coriander. Serve with basmati rice and coconut yogurt, if you like.
Per serving: 402 cals, 18g fat, 12g sat fat, 36g carbs

Baked sweet potatoes with cavolo nero and almonds

Tuck in to the comfort of a baked potato but with some tasty, healthy swaps

Serves 4 • Ready in 1 hr 30 mins

- 4 large sweet potatoes, washed
- 3tbsp olive oil
- 200g cavolo nero, roughly chopped
- 1 garlic clove, crushed
- 60g almonds
- houmous, to serve

1 Heat the oven to 200C/Gas 6. Rub the potatoes in 1tbsp oil and a pinch of sea salt. Wrap each one in foil, put into a roasting tin and bake for 1 hr 10 mins.
2 Spread out the cavolo nero in a large roasting tin. Sprinkle with the garlic and a little sea salt. Drizzle with 1tbsp oil, put in the oven and bake for 5 mins.
3 Scatter the almonds onto a baking tray, and sprinkle with a little sea salt and oil. Bake for 3 mins, to toast.
4 Cut each potato lengthways down the centre and squeeze the base to open up. Spoon in the cavolo nero and scatter over the almonds. Serve with houmous.
Per serving: 375 cals, 17g fat, 2g sat fat, 44g carbs

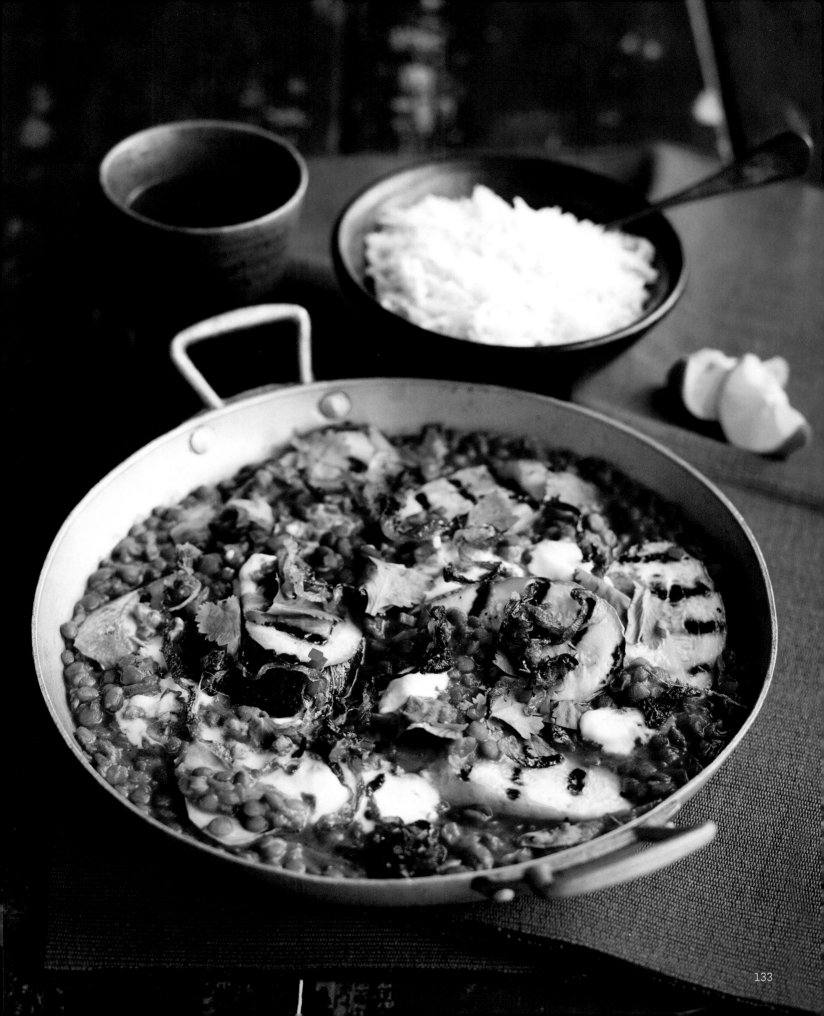

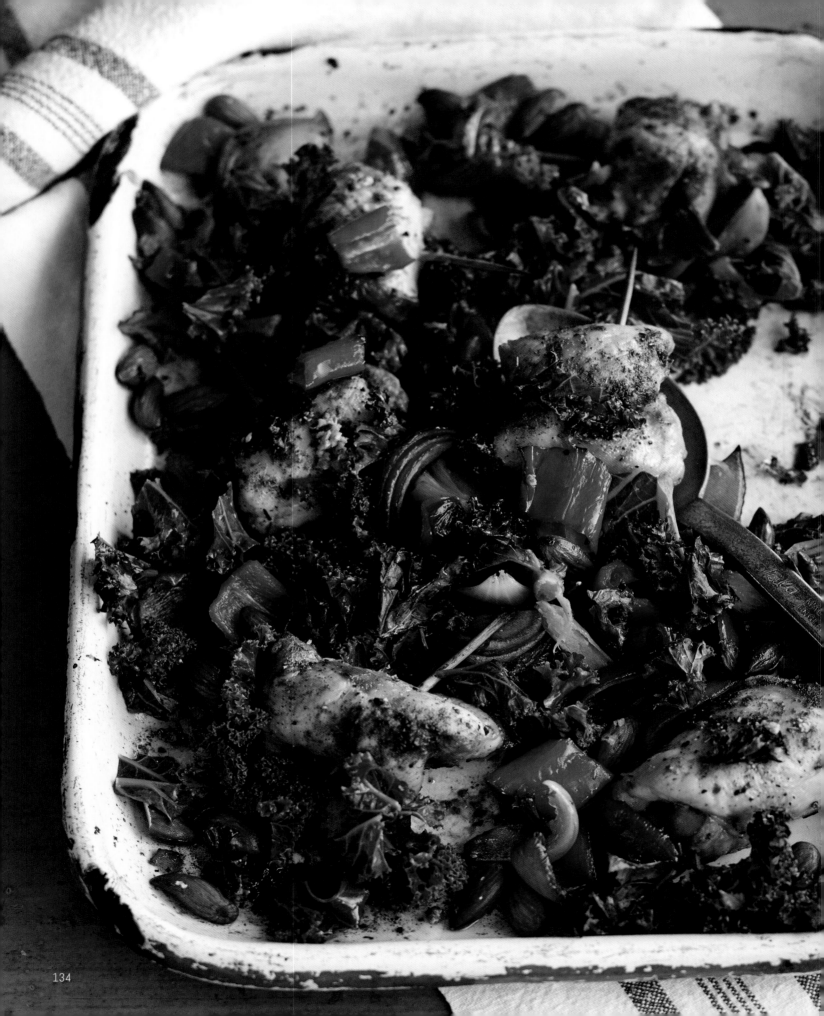

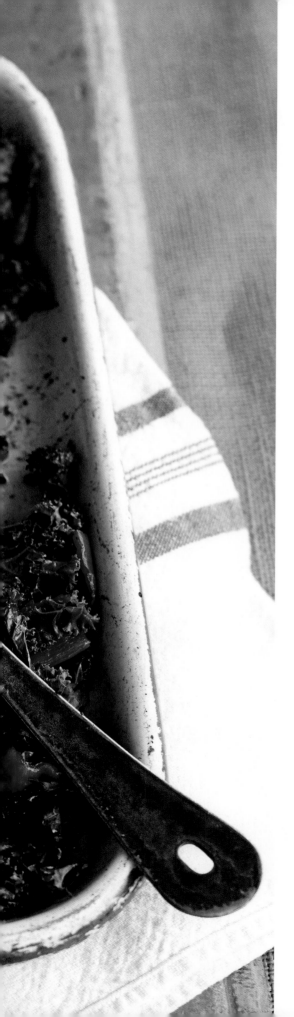

Health-boosting chicken and almond tray bake

High in protein, low in saturated fat and full of goodness, this tasty tray bake will become a favourite

Serves 2 • Ready in 40 mins

- 1tbsp barbecue seasoning
- 2 garlic cloves, crushed
- 6 skinless, boneless chicken thighs
- 3tbsp olive oil
- 2 red onions, cut into wedges
- 2 red peppers, deseeded and cubed
- 200g kale, chopped
- 60g whole almonds

1 Heat the oven to 200C/Gas 6. Sprinkle the barbecue seasoning and garlic over the chicken, then secure each piece into a neat shape with a cocktail stick.
2 Pour 1tbsp olive oil into the baking tray and arrange the chicken on top, along with the onions and peppers.
3 Drizzle 1tbsp oil over everything. Cook for 20 mins, until the chicken is browned.
4 Turn the chicken and vegetables, then add the kale and almonds. Sprinkle with a little sea salt and drizzle with the remaining oil. Cook for 5 mins, until the almonds are toasted and the kale is softened.
Per serving: 372 cals, 20g fat, 2g sat fat, 10.5g carbs

Health note

Just 30g of nuts a day, such as almonds, can help lower cholesterol.

Cauliflower and lentil curry

This takes the humble cauli to a new level; even committed meat-lovers won't complain!

Serves 4 • Ready in 50 mins

- 2tsp olive oil
- 400g can coconut milk
- 2 medium cauliflowers, trimmed and cut into florets
- 250g cooked puy lentils
- juice of 1 lemon
- 2tbsp freshly chopped coriander

For the paste:

- 2 garlic cloves, peeled
- 5cm piece root ginger, peeled and roughly chopped
- 1 green chilli
- 2 onions, very roughly chopped
- 1tbsp turmeric
- 1tbsp cumin
- 1tsp sea salt

1 For the paste, put all the ingredients into a blender and whizz to a paste. Heat the oil in a large saucepan, then gently fry the paste for a few mins to cook out the spices. Add the coconut milk, stir well, bring to the boil and simmer.

2 Meanwhile, steam or blanch the cauliflower florets until just tender, then add to the curry sauce. Simmer until just cooked and fully heated through, then add the puy lentils, lemon juice and coriander, and serve. This is great served with a tomato and onion salad, plus popadoms, naan breads or wholegrain rice.

Per serving: 390 cals, 25g fat, 16g sat fat, 24g carbs

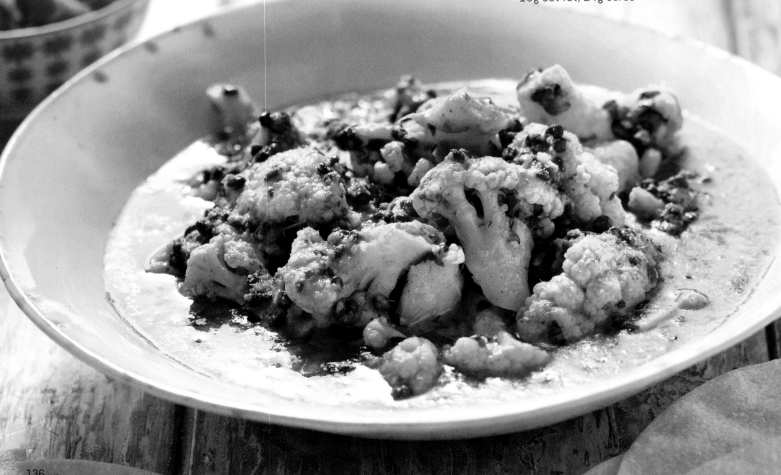

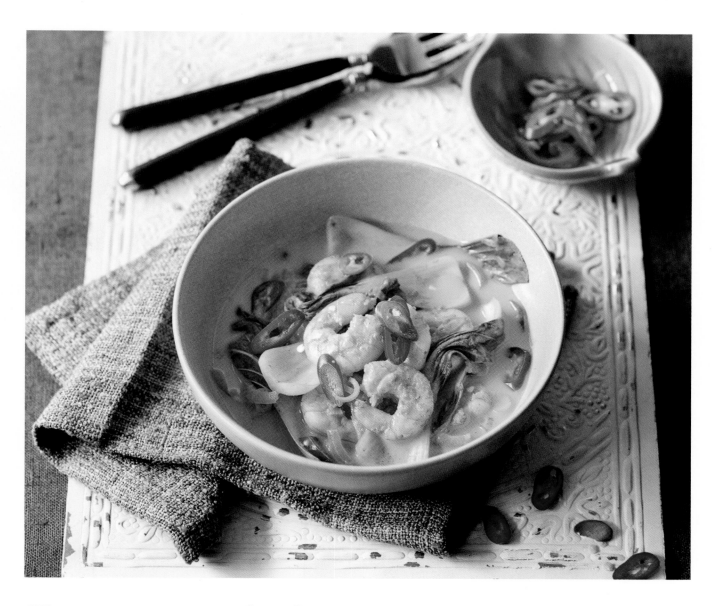

Vietnamese prawn broth

This restorative, flavour-packed broth takes just 15 mins to make and is ideal for a speedy, healthy midweek meal

Serves 2 • Ready in 15 mins

- 1tbsp olive oil
- 1 onion, thinly sliced
- 2 lemongrass sticks, trimmed and chopped
- 1-2 green chillies, deseeded and sliced
- 1-2tbsp curry powder
- 200ml semi-skimmed milk
- 1tsp sugar
- 1tbsp fish sauce
- 1tsp chicken stock powder
- 200g raw prawns
- 150g pak choi

1 Heat the oil in a pan and gently cook the onion, lemongrass, chillies and curry powder for about 5 mins, until softened and fragrant.

2 Add the milk, sugar, fish sauce, stock and prawns, then bring to a simmer. Cook for 3-4 mins until the prawns are just turning pink, then add the pak choi for 1-2 mins. Serve straight away, with extra chillies.
Per serving: 314 cals, 13.5g fat, 1.5g sat fat, 14g carbs

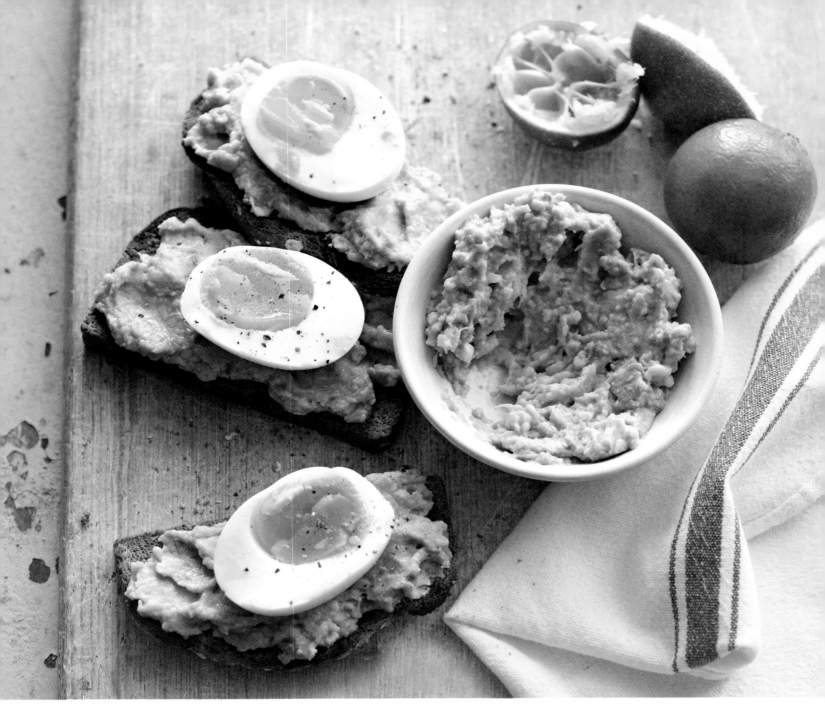

Smashed avo toast with soft-boiled eggs

Eggs are protein-rich and one of the few foods that contain vitamin D.
This dish will banish mid-morning munchies, too

Serves 4 • Ready in 15 mins

- 4 eggs
- 2 avocados
- juice of half a lime
- 8 slices of soda bread

1 Boil eggs in a pan of hot water for
7 mins to give a lightly-set centre.
Meanwhile, stone avocados and
peel and quarter them.
2 Put avocado flesh in a bowl and
season generously. Squeeze over
lime juice and mash well with a fork.

3 Toast soda bread slices and
peel eggs.
4 Spread mashed avocado on the
toast, halve the eggs then sit them
on top.
Per serving: 375 cals, 22g fat,
5g sat fat, 28g carbs

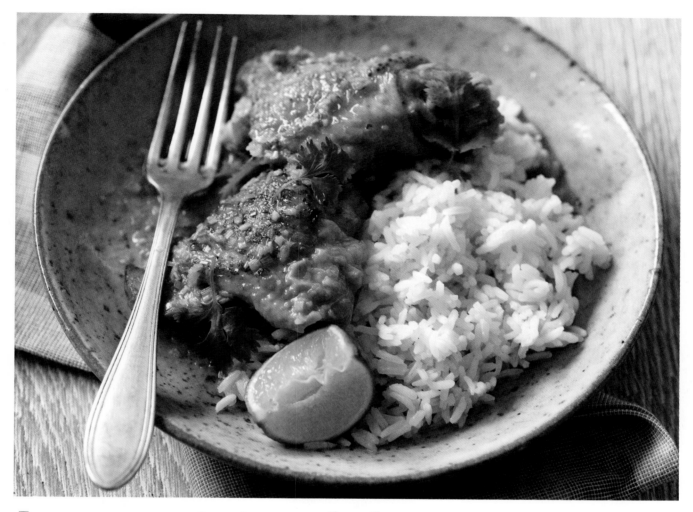

Lemongrass & ginger chicken

Lemongrass has long been used to ward off colds and fevers, and it combines well with the garlic and ginger. The chicken provides protein, B vitamins and selenium, which we need for a healthy immune system response

Serves 4 • Ready in 1 hr 40 mins

- 2tbsp fish sauce
- 1tbsp caster sugar
- 8 large chicken thighs
- 3 sticks lemongrass, finely sliced
- 3 garlic cloves, chopped
- 6cm fresh root ginger, peeled and chopped
- 2tbsp groundnut or other flavourless oil
- juice of a lime
- 2tbsp coriander, chopped

1 Mix fish sauce and sugar in a large bowl, then add chicken thighs, coating thoroughly in the mixture. Cover the chicken and place in the fridge to marinate for 30 mins.
2 Meanwhile blend sliced lemongrass, chopped garlic and ginger together in a food processor.
3 Heat oil in a large pan. Remove chicken from the marinade, add to the pan and brown well on all sides. Add lemongrass mixture and fry until fragrant.

4 Add marinade and 250ml water, stir well, cover and simmer over a low heat for 35 mins. Remove lid, add lime juice and chopped coriander, taste and adjust seasoning, serve with jasmine rice.
Per serving: 315 cals, 14g fat, 3g sat fat, 4g carbs

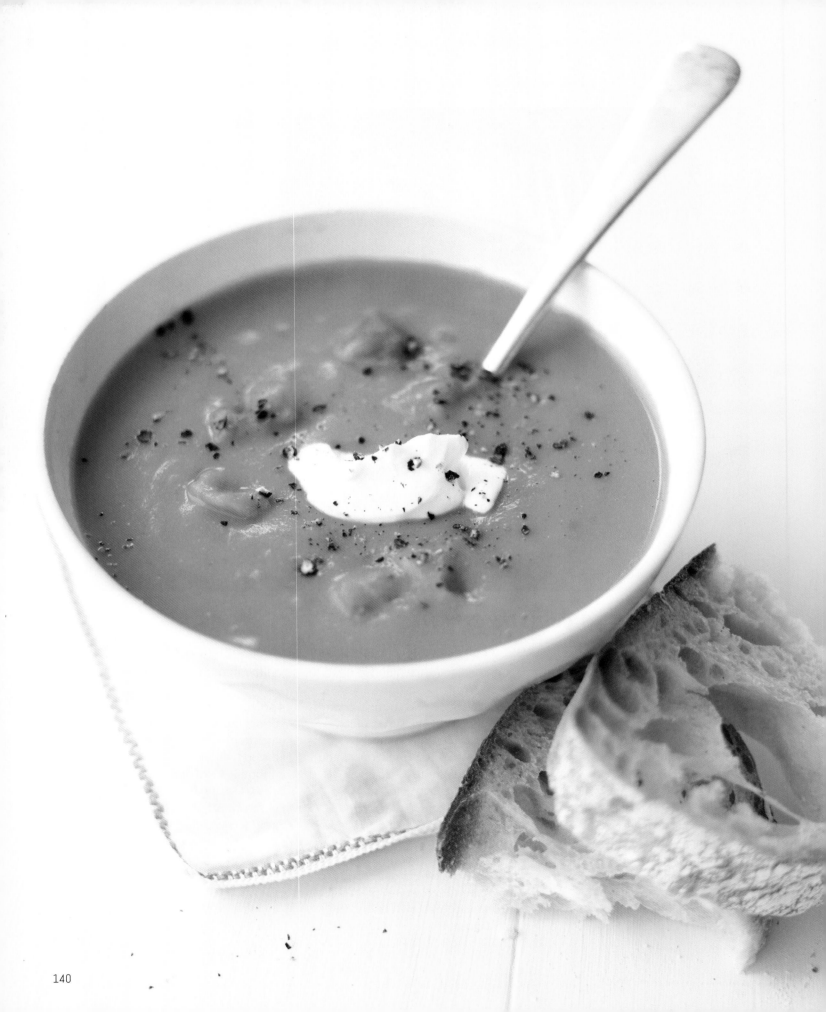

Spicy red pepper & lentil soup

This comforting soup is packed with vitamin C from the peppers, protein from the lentils and an immune-system boost from the garlic and chillies

Serves 4 • Ready in 40 mins

- 200g red lentils
- 2tbsp olive oil
- 1 medium onion, finely chopped
- 2 garlic cloves, peeled and crushed
- 1tsp crushed chillies
- 1tsp hot smoked paprika
- 4 red peppers, deseeded and diced
- 1litre vegetable stock
- 1tbsp sherry vinegar
- 1tsp caster sugar
- 4tbsp natural yogurt

1 Rinse red lentils, then leave to soak in cold water. In a large pan, warm olive oil and fry onion until soft. Add garlic and red chilli for 2 mins, then add sweet smoked paprika for a final min with a splash of water.
2 Add red peppers and cover for 10 mins, stirring occasionally. Drain lentils, add to the pan with the vegetable stock, cover, bring to the boil and simmer for 15 mins until lentils begin to break down.
3 Reserve a third of the soup and blend the rest. Stir back into the chunky soup, season to taste adding the sherry vinegar and caster sugar. Divide between 4 bowls and swirl 1tbsp natural yogurt through each.
Per serving: 293 cals, 7g fat, 1g sat fat, 38g carbs

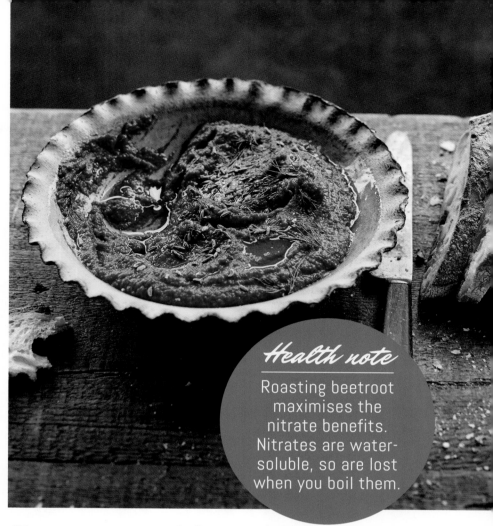

Health note

Roasting beetroot maximises the nitrate benefits. Nitrates are water-soluble, so are lost when you boil them.

Beetroot and fennel houmous

Beetroot is a bright choice in all ways – for colour, flavour and with nitrates for lowering blood pressure

Serves 4 • Ready in 50 mins

- 4 small beetroot
- 1 small fennel bulb, trimmed and tops reserved for garnish olive oil
- 1 tin organic chickpeas, drained and rinsed
- 1 fat garlic clove, peeled and crushed
- 1tsp fennel seeds, plus extra to garnish
- 1tbsp tahini
- generous squeeze of lemon juice
- 100-125ml extra virgin olive oil

1 Heat the oven to 200C/Gas 6. Wrap each beetroot individually in foil and put in a roasting tin. Slice the fennel and toss with a little oil in a separate small roasting tin, then season with freshly ground black pepper.
2 Put both tins in the oven and roast for 40 mins, until the fennel is softened and the beetroot is tender to the tip of a knife.
3 Once the beetroot are cool, peel them and put into a food processor with the roasted fennel, chickpeas, garlic, fennel seeds, tahini and lemon juice. Blitz to form a smooth paste, drizzling in the extra virgin olive oil as you go. Loosen with a little cold water if it is too thick. Garnish with fennel tops and fennel seeds.
Per serving: 254 cals, 21g fat, 3g sat fat, 14g carbs

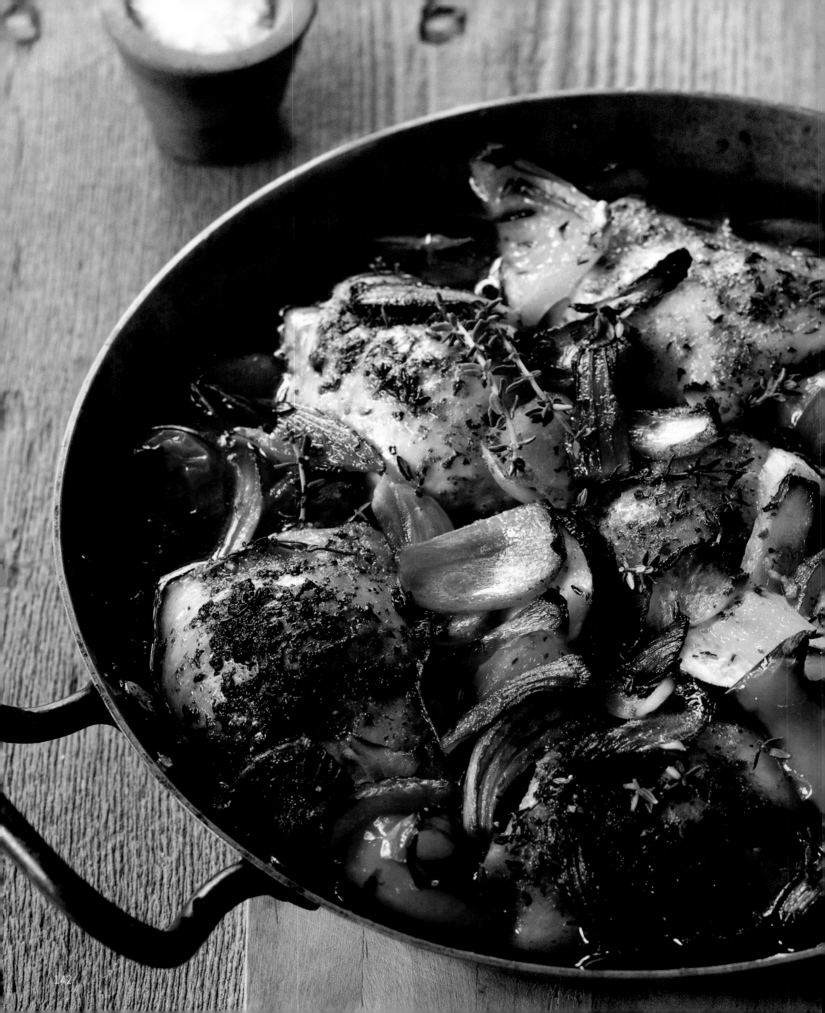

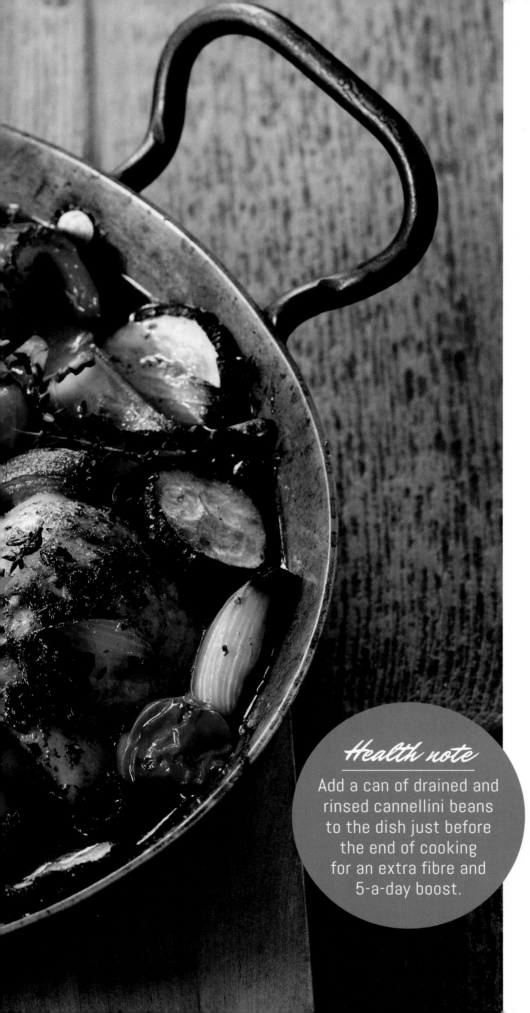

Zesty Mediterranean chicken

A fuss-free meal that is packed with fibre-rich vegetables

Serves 4 • Ready in 40 mins

- 6 chicken thighs
- 2tsp chicken seasoning
- 400g pack ready-to-roast
- Mediterranean vegetables (including onions, courgettes, peppers and cherry tomatoes)
- 2 garlic cloves, crushed
- juice of 2 lemons
- 2tbsp olive oil
- thyme sprigs, to serve (optional)
- extra salad or vegetables, to serve

1 Heat the oven to 200C/Gas 6. Put the chicken thighs in a large roasting tin and season with freshly ground black pepper and the chicken seasoning.
2 Add the Mediterranean vegetables and crushed garlic and pour over the lemon juice and olive oil.
3 Roast in the oven for 30–35 mins until the chicken is golden and cooked through and the vegetables are tender. Scatter with thyme sprigs, to serve.
Per serving: 345 cals, 19g fat, 4g sat fats, 7g carbs

Health note

Add a can of drained and rinsed cannellini beans to the dish just before the end of cooking for an extra fibre and 5-a-day boost.

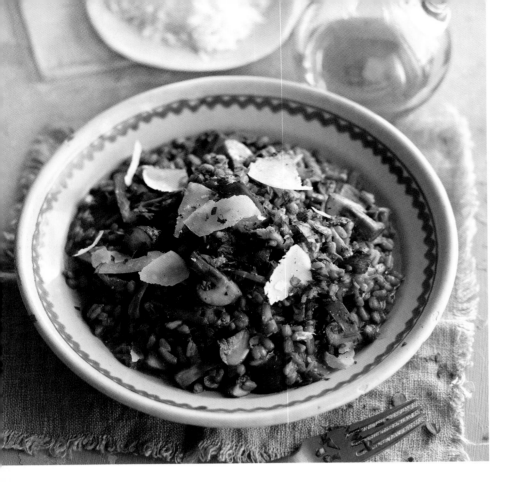

Mixed mushrooms and spelt

Spelt is an ancient grain that is high in fibre and nutrients linked to a reduced risk of heart disease

Serves 6 • Ready in 40 mins

- 2tbsp olive oil, plus extra
- 1 large onion, chopped
- 1 stick celery, chopped
- 1 carrot peeled and chopped
- 2 garlic cloves
- 200g chestnut mushrooms, chopped
- 350g spelt
- 200ml red wine
- 1.2 litres low-salt hot beef stock
- 100g pack wild mushrooms
- Parmesan shavings and chopped parsley, to garnish

1 Heat the oil and cook the onion, celery, carrot and garlic for 10 mins. Add the chestnut mushrooms and cook for a further 2 mins. Stir in the spelt, then add the wine. Cook until the wine has absorbed. Add the stock and simmer for 25 mins, or until the spelt is tender.
2 Fry the wild mushrooms in a little oil and add to the spelt mixture, along with the Parmesan shavings and the fresh parsley.
Per serving 191 cals per serving, 5g fat, 1g sat fat, 23g carbs

Health note

Onions contain quercetin that can also help reduce blood pressure.

Sweet potato, squash and lentil casserole

A delicious, subtly spiced low-fat but hearty meat-free dinner

Serves 4 • Ready in 45 mins

- 1tbsp olive oil
- 2 celery sticks, thinly sliced
- 1 onion, chopped
- 2 garlic cloves, roughly chopped
- 350g mix of sweet potato and butternut squash, cut into bite-sized pieces
- 1 Granny Smith apple, peeled and chopped
- 1tbsp medium curry powder
- 100g red lentils, rinsed
- 1 vegetable stock cube
- 1tbsp tomato purée
- 1tbsp mango chutney
- fresh coriander leaves, to garnish

1 Heat the oil in a large pan and cook the celery, onion and garlic for 8–10 mins, until beginning to soften.
2 Add the sweet potato and butternut squash to the pan along with the apple, curry powder and lentils. Cook, stirring, for a further 2 mins. Add 650ml hot water to the pan with the stock cube, tomato purée and mango chutney. Bring to the boil, then reduce the heat and simmer gently for around 25 mins, until the vegetables and lentils are tender. Serve ladled into deep bowls, garnished with coriander leaves.
Per serving: 219 cals, 4g fat, 0.5g saturated, 36g carbs

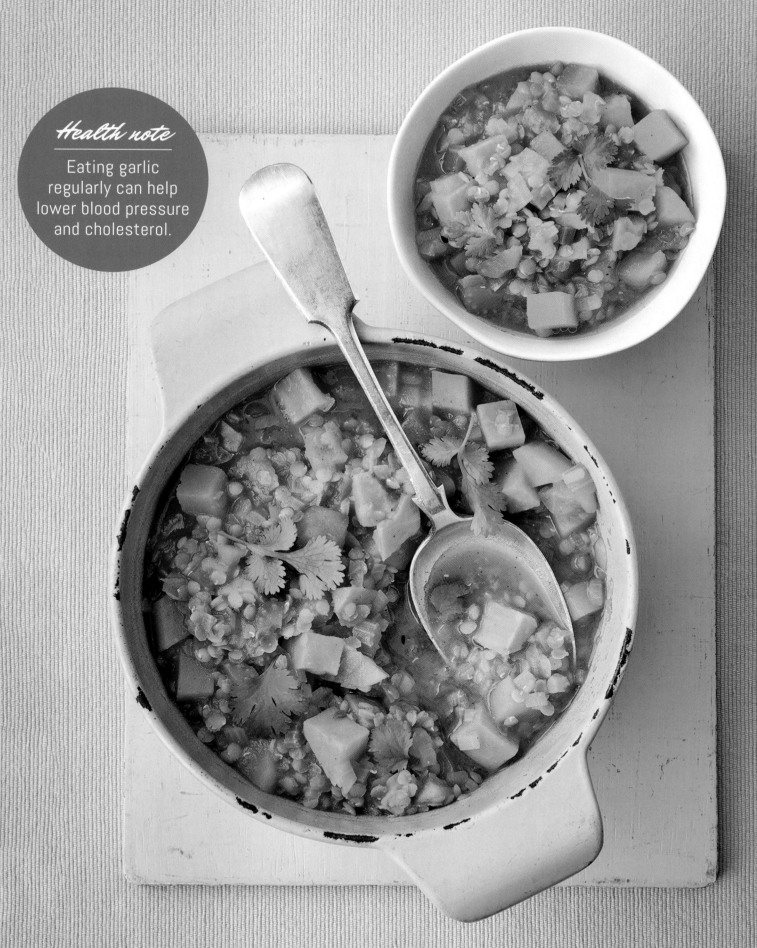

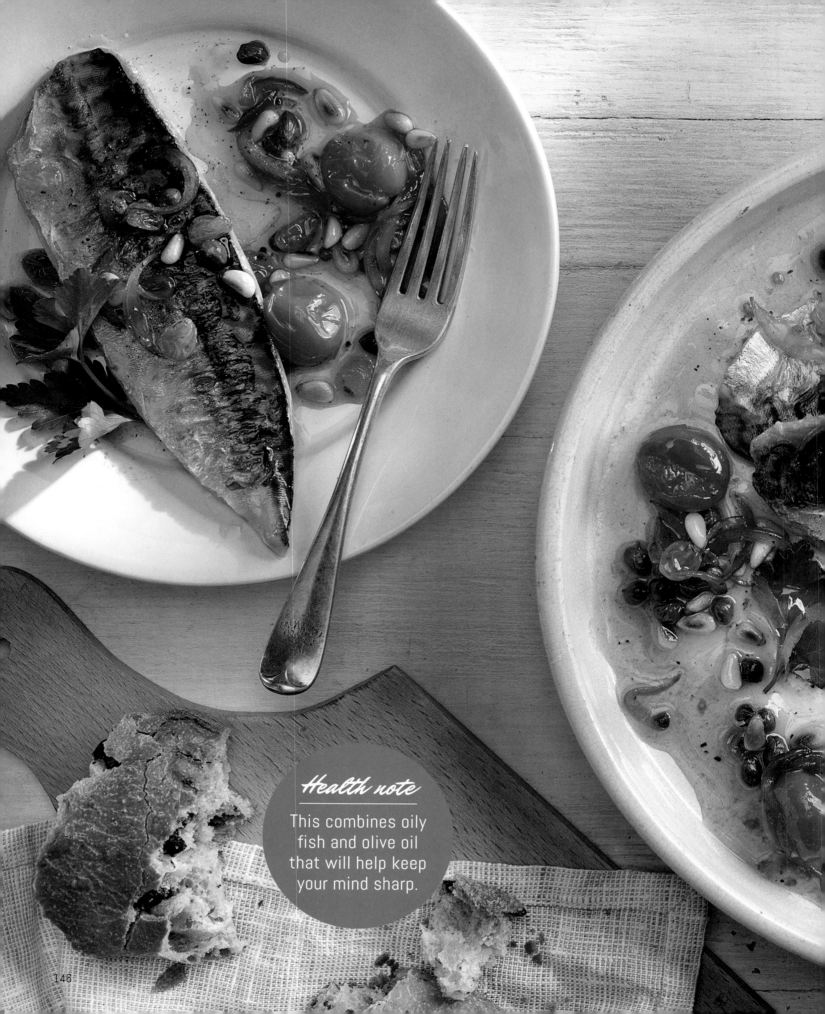

Health note

This combines oily fish and olive oil that will help keep your mind sharp.

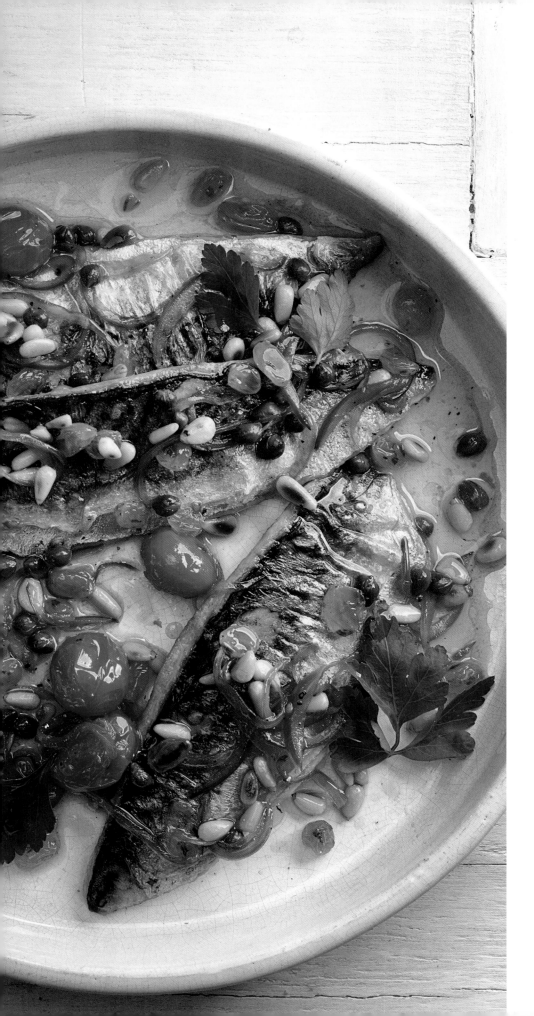

Sicilian-style mackerel

A delicious recipe of light and fresh-tasting fresh mackerel

Serves 4 • Ready in 25 mins

- 5tbsp extra virgin olive oil
- 4 large or 8 small, very fresh mackerel fillets
- 1 small red onion, halved and finely sliced
- 200g cherry tomatoes
- 1 garlic clove, sliced
- 3tbsp red wine vinegar
- 2½tbsp caster sugar
- 1 heaped tbsp capers, rinsed and drained
- 2tbsp golden raisins or sultanas
- 2tbsp pine nuts, toasted
- handful of flat-leaf parsley leaves
- crusty bread, to serve

1 Put 2tbsp of the olive oil in a large frying pan set over a medium-high heat. Add the mackerel fillets, skin-side down, and sear for 2 mins, until the skin is golden and crisp.
2 Carefully turn over the fish, cook for 1-2 mins, depending on size, then remove to a plate and set aside. Turn the heat down a little, add the onion and cook, stirring often, for 5 mins. Stir in the tomatoes and garlic, and cook for a further 2 mins. Add the red wine vinegar, sugar, capers, raisins and pine nuts and simmer for 1 min or so. Season to taste, then return the fish to the pan. Warm through, then drizzle with the remaining olive oil and scatter the parsley over. Serve with the crusty bread.
Per serving: 613 cals, 46g fat, 8g sat fat, 19g carbs

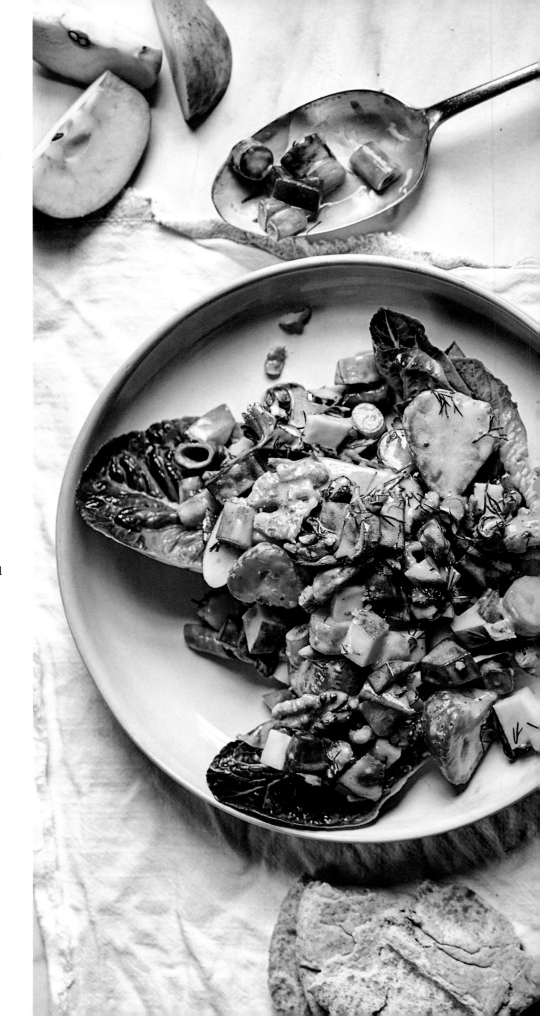

Waldorf salad

A simple assembly job salad that ticks a lot of brain-friendly boxes

Serves 6 • Ready in 15 mins

- 100g walnut pieces
- 2 baby leaf lettuces
- 45g baby leaf spinach leaves
- 45g rocket
- 16 radishes, cut in half
- 100g cooked beetroot, chopped
- 2 carrots, finely chopped
- 6 spring onions, roughly chopped
- 45g raisins
- 2 apples, cored and cut into small pieces
- 200g strawberries, halved
- large handful flat-leaf parsley, roughly chopped

For the dressing:
- 100ml olive oil
- 100ml cider vinegar
- 200g natural yogurt
- 1tbsp tahini
- 2tsp wholegrain mustard
- handful fresh dill, roughly chopped

1 In a small frying pan, toast the walnuts over a medium heat for 2 mins, until golden. Set aside.
2 Combine the dressing ingredients.
3 Arrange the lettuce, spinach and rocket in 6 flat bowls. Put the remaining ingredients, reserving half the parsley, into a mixing bowl. Pour over the dressing and carefully mix to combine.
4 Divide the salad between the 6 bowls. Use the remainder of the parsley and almonds to garnish.
Per serving 389 cals, 27g fat, 4g sat fat, 26g carbs

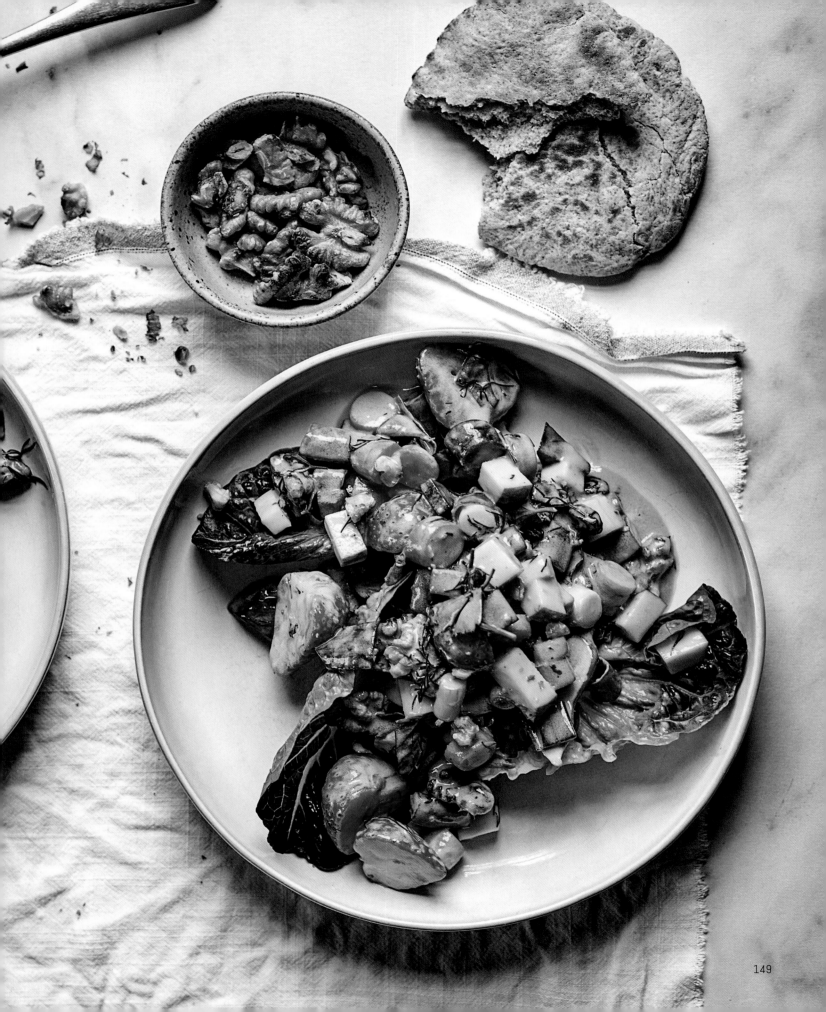

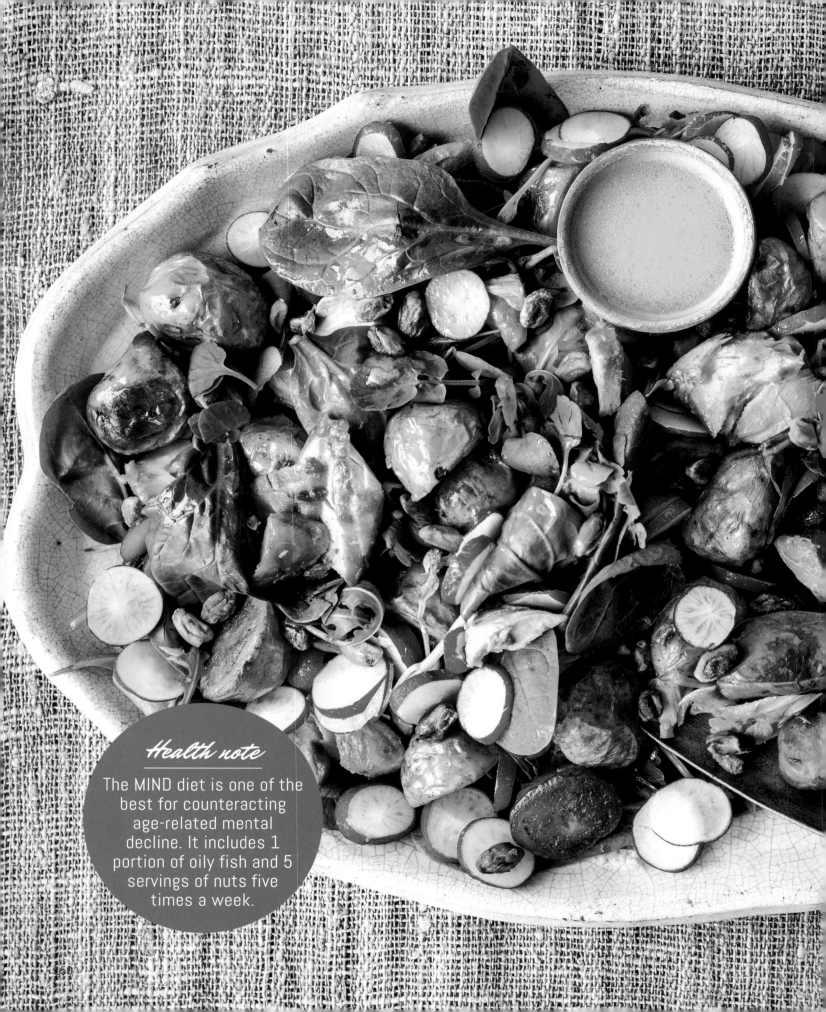

Health note

The MIND diet is one of the best for counteracting age-related mental decline. It includes 1 portion of oily fish and 5 servings of nuts five times a week.

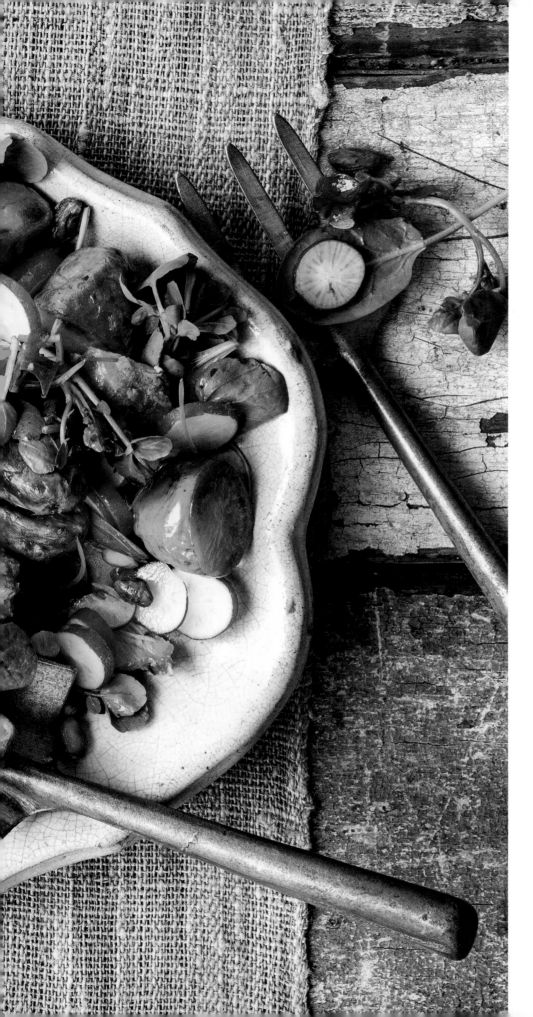

Roasted new potato and salmon salad

A satisfying salad with a helping of salmon that is a source of omega-3 fatty acids

Serves 4 • Ready in 40 mins

- 500g baby new potatoes, halved
- 1 garlic clove, crushed
- 2tbsp olive oil
- 100g pistachios, shelled
- ¼tsp sea salt
- 125g watercress, rocket and spinach mixed salad
- 200g hot-smoked salmon, flaked
- 200g radishes, trimmed and sliced

For the dressing:
- 2tbsp olive oil
- 1tbsp white wine vinegar
- 1tbsp maple syrup
- 1tsp Dijon mustard

1 Heat the oven to 220C/Gas 7. Arrange the potatoes in a tin with the garlic and oil and roast for 30 mins, until they are tender and golden.

2 Spread the pistachios onto a baking tray, scatter with sea salt and 3tbsp water. Cook in the oven for 3–5 mins, until the nuts are toasted.

3 Arrange the salad on a platter. Top with the pistachios, salmon and radishes. Put the dressing ingredients in a lidded jar with 2tbsp water and season. Shake. Serve with the salad.

Per serving: 470 cals, 5g fat, 2g sat fat, 25g carbs

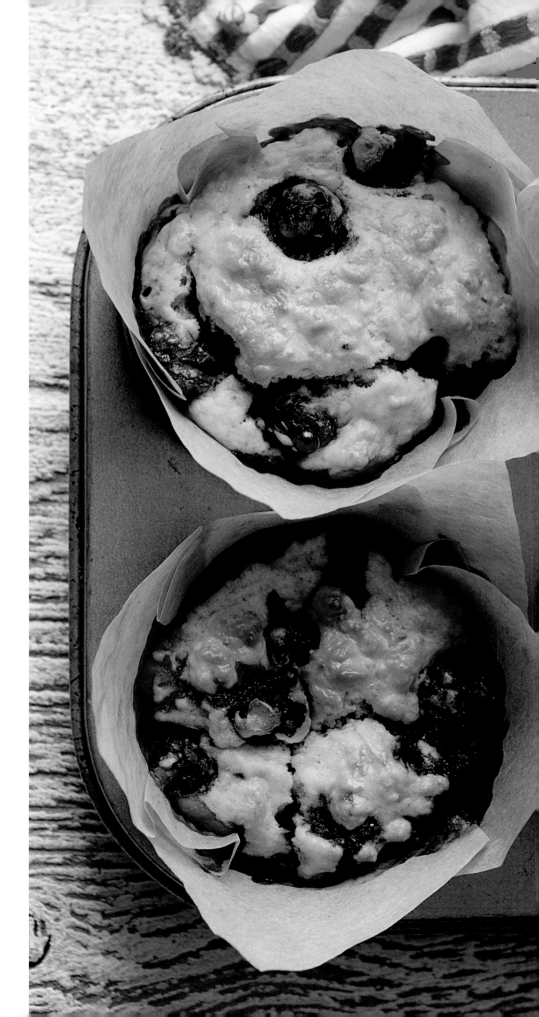

Healthy blueberry muffins

These tasty, dairy-free muffins use natural fats and sweeteners, which are good for both body and mind

Makes 6 • Ready in 30 mins

- 150g self-raising flour
- 1tsp baking powder
- 2-4tbsp stevia sweetener (e.g. Truvia)
- 160ml can coconut cream
- 2 medium eggs
- 4tbsp nut or soy milk
- 200g punnet blueberries

You will need:
- 6-hole muffin tin with paper cases

1 1 Heat the oven to 200C/Gas 6.
2 Sift the flour and baking powder into a bowl. Stir in the sweetener. Tip the coconut cream into a jug, then beat in the eggs and milk, until smooth. Pour the mixture into the flour, add the blueberries and stir until just mixed. Divide the mixture between the lined muffin cases.
3 Bake for 15–20 mins, or until risen and just firm to the touch in the centre. Remove from the oven and place them on a wire rack to cool.
Per serving: 193 cals, 8.5g fat, 5.5g sat fat, 24g carbs

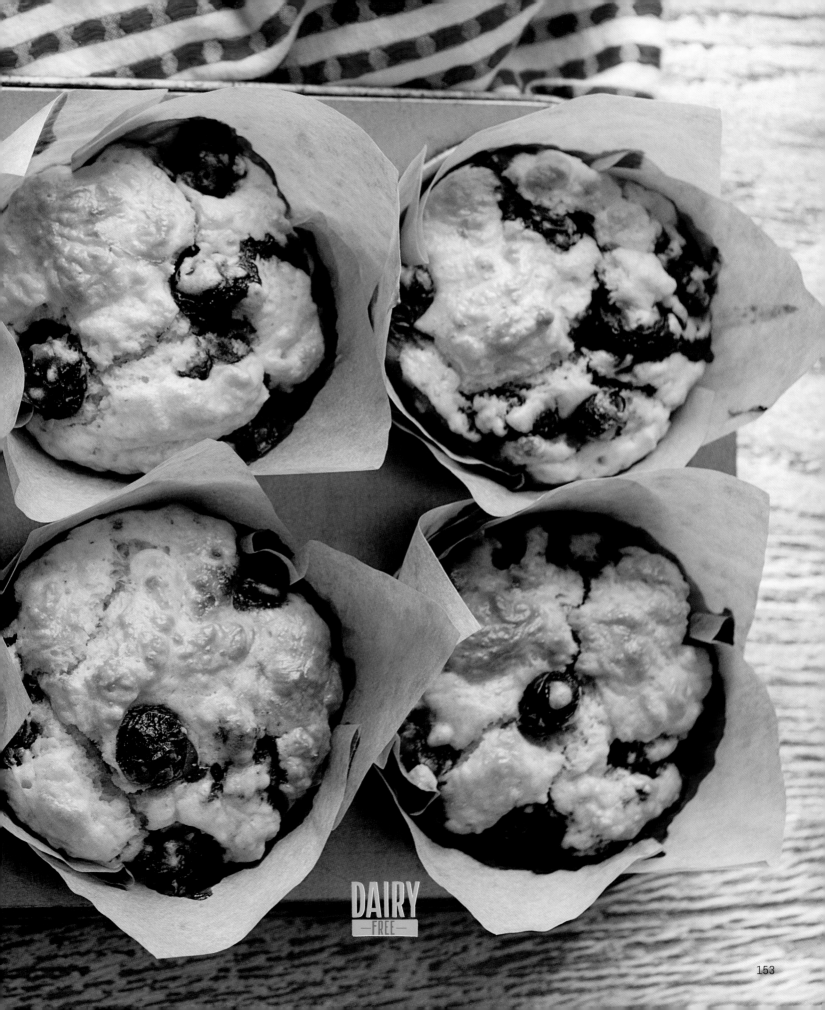

Raspberry polenta cake

This cake is easy to make but looks and tastes gorgeous. Serve with a cup of tea

Serves 8 • Ready in 1 hr 20 mins, plus cooling

- 125g caster sugar
- 3 eggs, separated
- 175ml olive oil
- Zest and juice of 1 orange
- 225g fine polenta
- 60g ground almonds
- 1½tsp gluten-free baking powder
- 150g raspberries
- 1 peach, cut into pieces
- 15g flaked almonds
- 1tbsp honey
- juice of 1 lemon

You will need:
- 20cm cake tin, the base lined and greased

1 Heat the oven to 180C/Gas 4. Whisk the sugar and egg yolks until thick and pale. Slowly incorporate the oil and orange juice while whisking.
2 Mix the polenta, ground almonds, baking powder and orange zest into the egg yolk mixture.
3 Whisk the egg whites until stiff and fold in a third at a time, until well combined. Put the mixture into the tin, and top with the raspberries, peach and flaked almonds.
4 Bake for 50 mins, until a cocktail stick inserted in the top comes out clean. Cool in the tin for 5 mins, then transfer to a cooling rack.
5 Meanwhile, warm the honey and lemon juice, stirring to dissolve the honey, and set aside to cool. While the cake is still warm, drizzle or brush the honey mixture over the top.
Per serving: 242 cals, 24g fat, 3g sat fat, 42g carbs

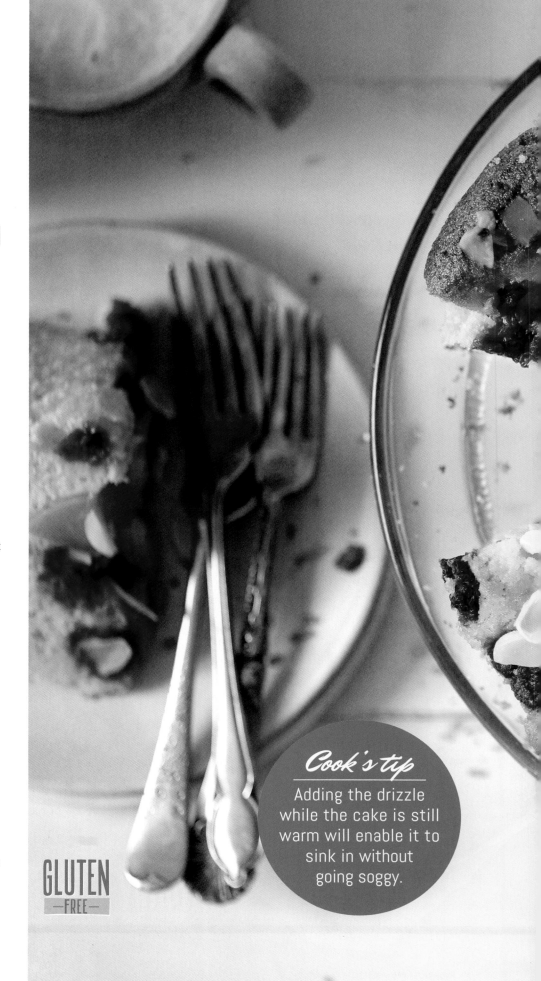

GLUTEN
—FREE—

Cook's tip
Adding the drizzle while the cake is still warm will enable it to sink in without going soggy.

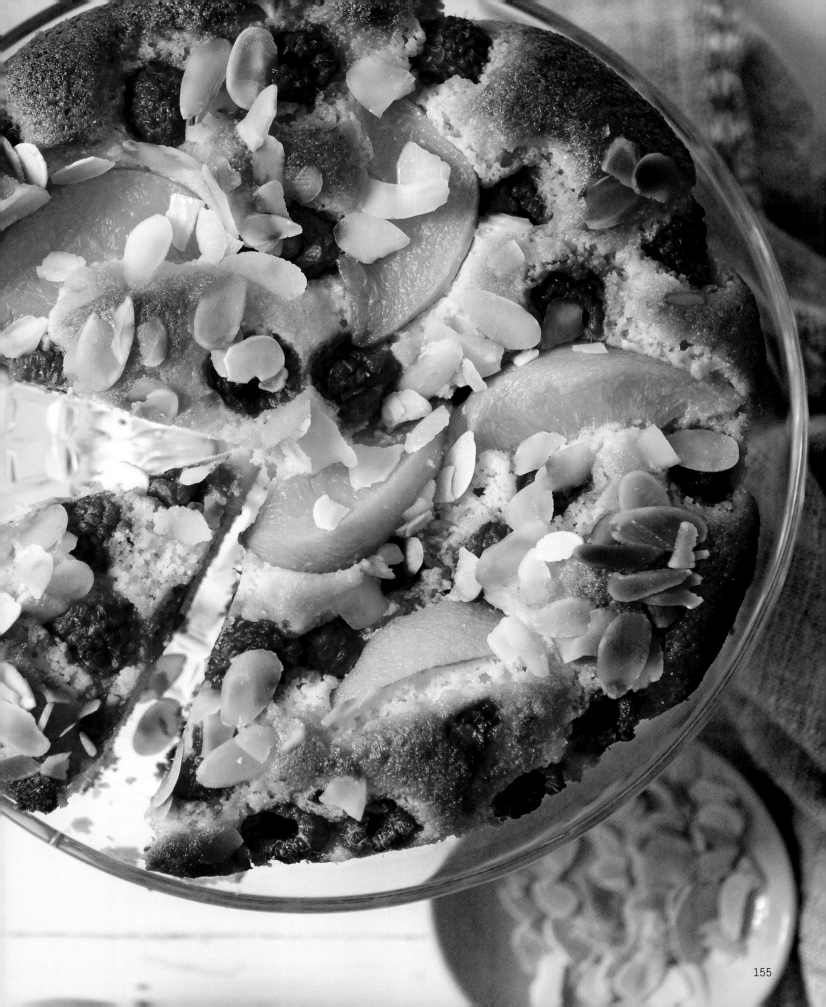

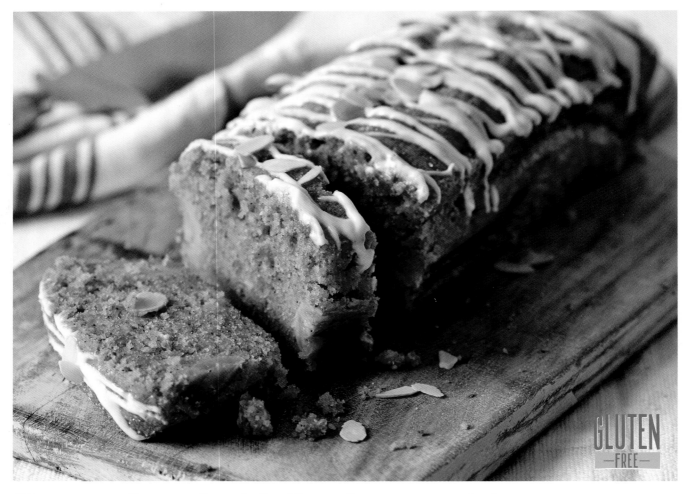

GLUTEN
—FREE—

Banana bread with Greek yogurt icing

Lightly spiced and bursting with banana, this makes the ultimate breakfast served with a dollop of Greek yogurt

Serves 10 • Ready in 1 hr, plus cooling

- 225g very ripe bananas
- pinch ground clove, to taste
- 150g unsalted butter
- 150g caster sugar
- 2 eggs
- 150g gluten-free plain flour
- 1tsp gluten-free baking powder
- 45g ground almonds
- 1½tsp cinnamon
- toasted flaked almonds, to decorate

For the yogurt glaze:
- 75g 0% fat Greek-style yogurt
- 15g icing sugar
- ½tsp almond extract

You will need:
- 10x25cm loaf tin, greased and lined

1 Heat the oven to 160C/Gas 3. Slice 1 of the bananas in half lengthways, set aside, then mash the rest in a bowl with the ground clove.

2 In another bowl, cream the butter and sugar together until light and fluffy. Mix in the eggs, flour, baking powder, ground almonds and cinnamon until you have a smooth batter. Fold through the mashed banana.

3 Place the sliced banana halves against the side of your loaf tin. Pour in the cake batter then bake for 40-45 mins until a skewer comes out clean.

4 Whisk together the yogurt glaze ingredients to combine then chill until the cake is completely cool. Drizzle the glaze over the cake and top with the toasted flaked almonds.

Per serving: 283 cals, 15g fat, 8g sat fat, 31g carbs

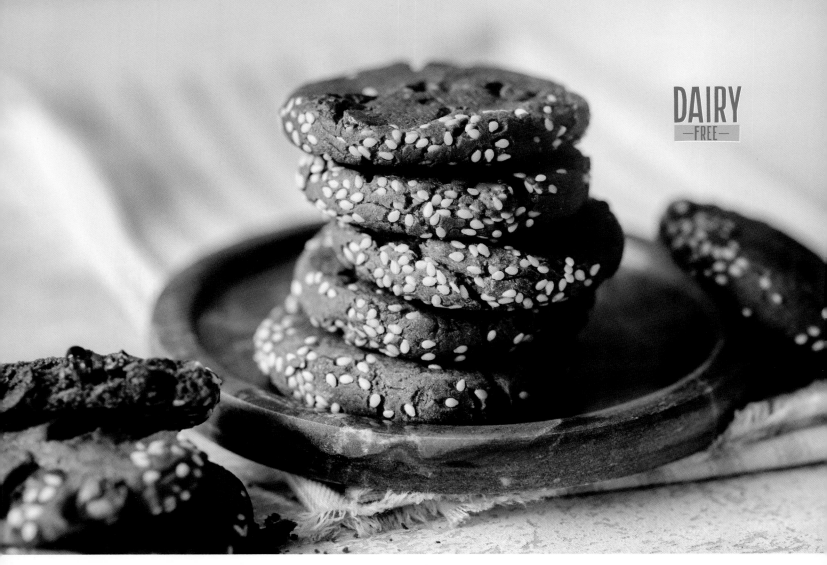

Chocolate chip tahini cookies

These combine rich, dark chocolate chips with the nutty flavour of tahini to create a complex, tasty and well-balanced flavour

Serves 24 • Ready in 45 mins, plus chilling

- 100g dairy-free butter, softened
- 175g light brown soft sugar
- 1 egg
- 60g tahini
- 200g plain flour
- 1tsp baking powder
- 4tbsp cocoa powder
- 100g dark chocolate chips or roughly chopped dark chocolate
- 75g sesame seeds

1 In a large bowl, beat the dairy-free butter and sugar until creamy, then gradually beat in the egg and the tahini. Sift the flour, baking powder and cocoa powder over the mixture and stir to combine, then mix in the chocolate chips. Once the dough comes together, tip out onto a clean surface and knead into a 24cm cylindrical log.
2 Sprinkle the sesame seeds onto a chopping board and roll the dough so the seeds stick and cover the outside. When the edges are covered in seeds, wrap the dough

in cling film and chill in the fridge for 1 hr.
3 Heat the oven to 180C/Gas 4. Remove the dough from the fridge and, using a sharp knife, cut it into 1cm discs. Place on a baking tray lined with parchment, leaving a space between the cookies.
4 Bake the cookies for 10-12 mins until cooked through. Remove from the oven and allow to cool completely on a rack before serving.
Per serving: 154 cals, 8.5g fat, 3.5g sat fat, 15g carbs

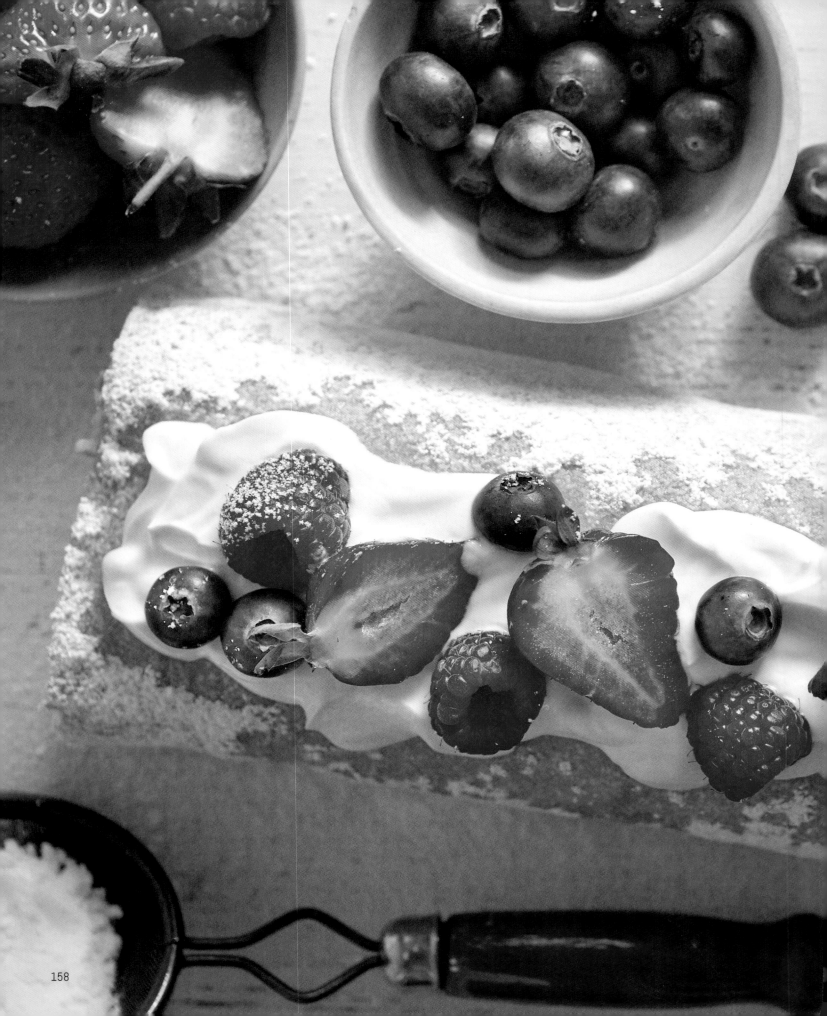

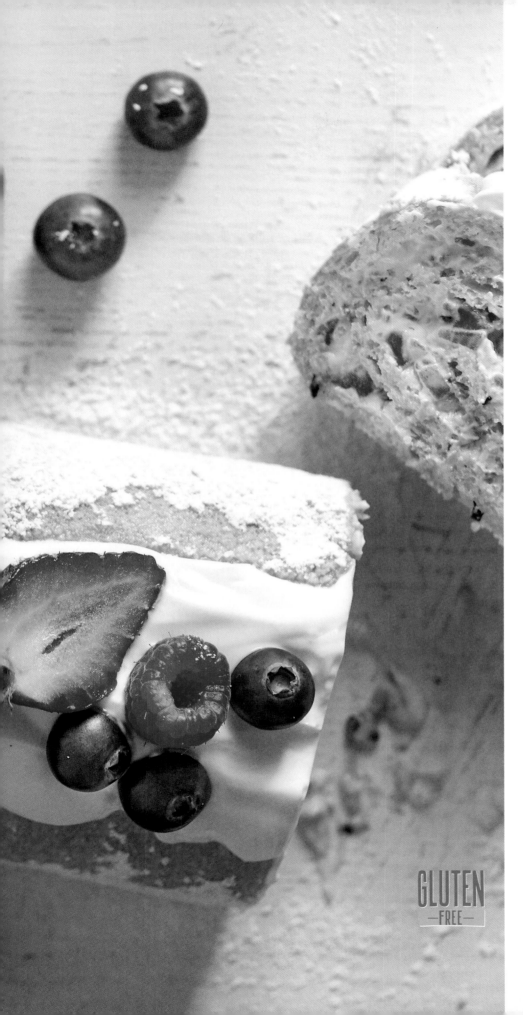

Summer fruit roulade

This is low in fat and bursting with berries, and makes a great centrepiece for when friends or family are over

Serves 12 • Ready in 40 mins, plus cooling

- 5 eggs, 4 of them separated
- 115g caster sugar
- 75g ground almonds
- 1tbsp cornflour
- 2tbsp icing sugar

For the filling:
- 150g mixed berries, chopped, plus extra for garnish
- 300g 0% fat Greek yogurt, plus extra for topping

You will need:
- 39x24cm Swiss roll tin, lined with parchment

1 Heat the oven to 160C/Gas 3. Whisk 4 egg whites in the bowl of a standing mixer. Gradually add 45g of the caster sugar, 1tbsp at a time, until stiff peaks begin to form.

2 In a different bowl, whisk together the whole egg and 2 egg yolks with the remaining 70g sugar and the ground almonds until doubled in size.

3 Fold a third of the whisked egg whites into the eggs and almonds to lighten, followed by the remaining two-thirds. Sift in the cornflour and gently fold together. Pour into the Swiss roll tin, level with a palette knife and bake for 3–4 mins, or until lightly golden.

4 Remove from the oven and cool in the tin for a few mins before turning onto a piece of parchment dusted with icing sugar. Leave to cool further.

5 Mix the chopped berries with the yogurt and spread over the sponge. With the shortest side of the sponge facing you, roll the roulade. Place on a board, top with more yogurt and berries, and serve.

Per serving: 150 cals, 6g fat, 1g sat fat, 15g carbs

GLUTEN
—FREE—

Elderflower cheesecake

This dairy-free version is perfect for those with food intolerances, but tastes so good that everyone will love it!

Serves 12 • Ready in 1 hr 15 mins, plus cooling and overnight chilling

For the base:
- 150g dairy-, wheat- and gluten-free digestive biscuits
- 45g olive oil spread

For the filling:
- 750g dairy-free cream cheese
- 175g golden caster sugar
- 254g carton single soya 10% fat
- 2tbsp gluten-free cornflour
- 1tbsp vanilla bean paste
- finely grated zest and juice of 1 lemon
- 3tbsp elderflower cordial
- 2 eggs

For the topping:
- 4tbsp elderflower cordial

You will need:
- edible flowers, such as violas or elderflowers (optional)
- 18cm springform tin, greased and lined

1 Heat the oven to 180C/Gas 4. For the base, blitz the biscuits in a food processor to make crumbs. Melt the olive oil spread in the microwave, add to the crumbs and mix. Press into the base of the tin and bake for 10 mins, then cool.

2 For the filling, put the dairy-free cream cheese, sugar and single soya into a food processor and blend to combine. Stir the cornflour with 4tbsp water until dissolved and add to the dairy-free cream cheese mix with the vanilla, lemon zest and juice, cordial and eggs. Blend the mixture until smooth and creamy.

3 Pour the mixture over the biscuit base and place the cake tin in a roasting tin. Pour boiling water around the cake tin to come halfway up the tin. Cook for 10 mins. Reduce the oven temperature to 160C/Gas 3 and bake for 35 mins. Leave in the oven for 1 hr, then cool and chill overnight.

4 For the topping, heat the cordial for a few mins until it turns pale golden, then immediately drizzle it over the top of the cheesecake. Decorate with edible flowers, if you like.

Per serving: 460 cals, 31g fat, 5g sat fat, 30g carbs

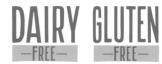

DAIRY
—FREE—
GLUTEN
—FREE—

Cook's tip
Try using the zest or juice of a lime instead of a lemon for a different flavour profile.

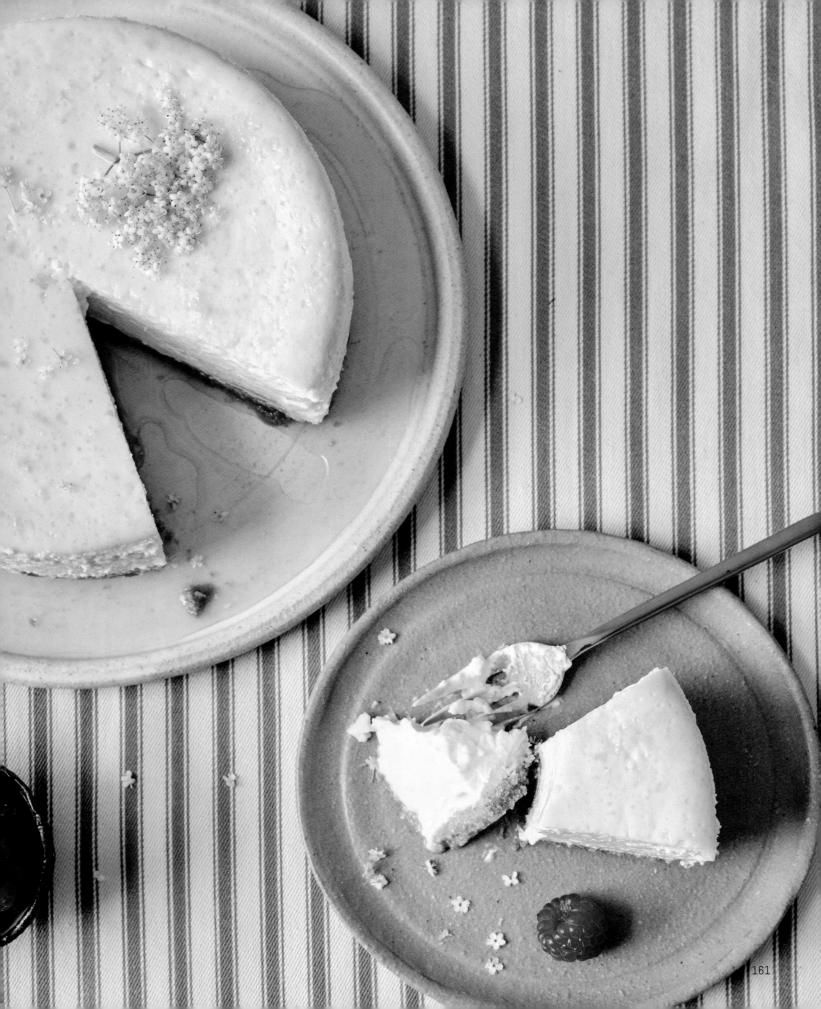

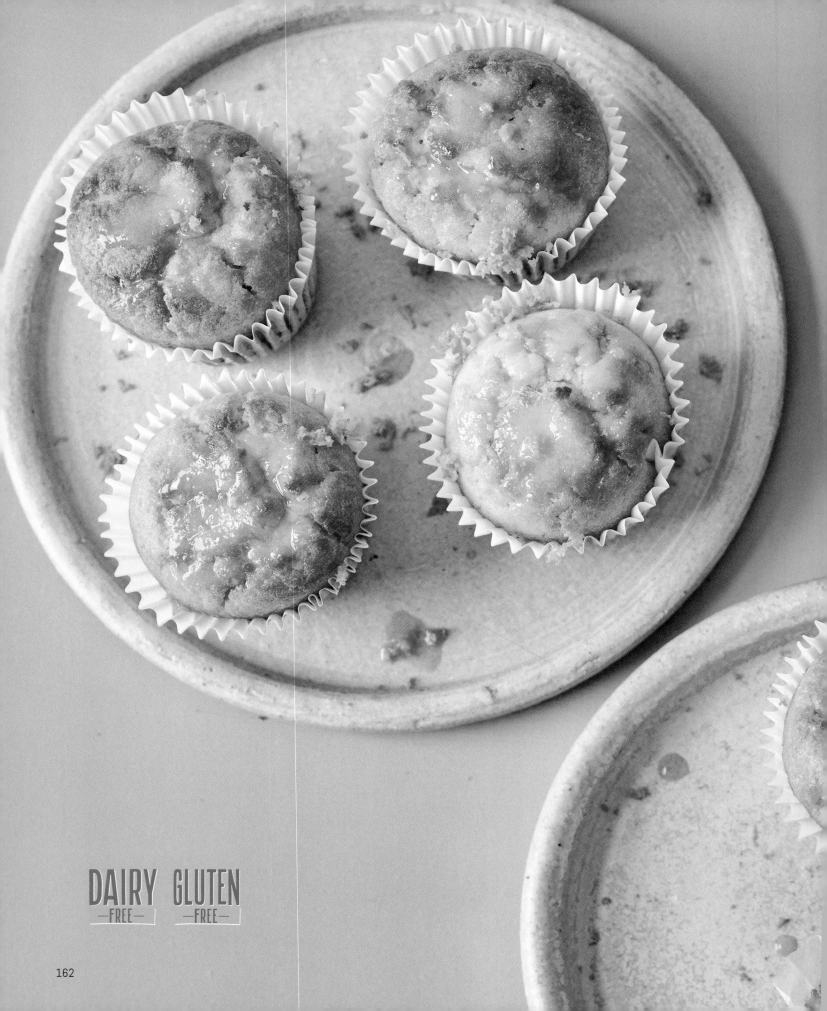

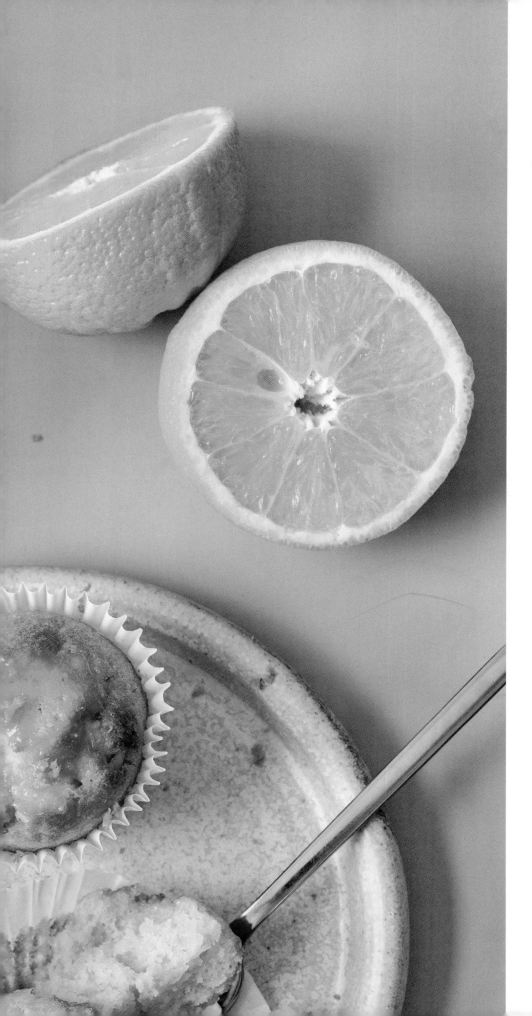

Orange fairy cakes

These individual cakes are infused with a fresh, citrus orange flavour, and are perfect for elevenses

Makes 8 • Ready in 30 mins, plus cooling

- 125g gluten-free plain white flour
- 1 level tsp gluten-free baking powder
- 125g dairy-free spread
- 90g Fruisana fruit sugar (or 125g caster sugar), plus 1 extra tbsp
- 2 eggs
- grated rind and juice of 1 large orange

You will need:
- 8-hole muffin tin, lined with paper cases

1 Heat the oven to 190C/Gas 5. Put the flour, baking powder, spread, 90g sugar and the eggs in a mixing bowl, and add half the orange rind and 1tbsp water. Beat well with a wooden spoon until mixed. Spoon the mixture into the paper cake cases and bake for 15 mins.
2 Remove the cakes from the muffin tin and place on a wire rack to cool.
3 Heat the orange juice in a small pan with 1tbsp water and the extra 1tbsp sugar. Boil until syrupy. Pour over the hot fairy cakes, then sprinkle with the rest of the grated orange rind. Leave the fairy cakes to cool before serving.
Per serving: 260 cals, 15g fat, 7g sat fat, 32g carbs

Raspberry and coconut ice cream

A vegan and naturally sweetened ice cream that's refreshing and light

- 100g pitted Medjool dates
- 250g raspberries
- 2 x 400ml tins coconut milk, chilled overnight in the fridge
- 1tsp cornflour

You will need:

- 450g loaf tin

1 Soak the Medjool dates in 100ml boiling water for 10 mins. Remove 2tbsp of the water and set it aside. Then blend the dates and water in a food processor until smooth. Add the raspberries and a pinch of salt and blend again.

2 Scoop the hardened coconut cream that's at the top of the tins out into a bowl and whisk for 5 mins until fluffy. Mix the cornflour with the 2tbsp reserved water and add to the coconut with the raspberry mix. Whisk until combined and thickened, and place in the loaf tin. Cover with baking parchment and freeze for 1 hr.

3 Remove from the freezer and blend in a food processor until smooth. Return the mixture to the freezer for 1 hr then blend again. Pour back into the tin, cover with baking parchment once more and freeze overnight. Leave at room temperature for 5 mins before serving with fresh raspberries, if you like.

Per serving: 380 cals, 29g fat, 24g sat fat, 32g carbs

Cook's tip
Try this recipe with the same quantity of another berry.

DAIRY
—FREE—

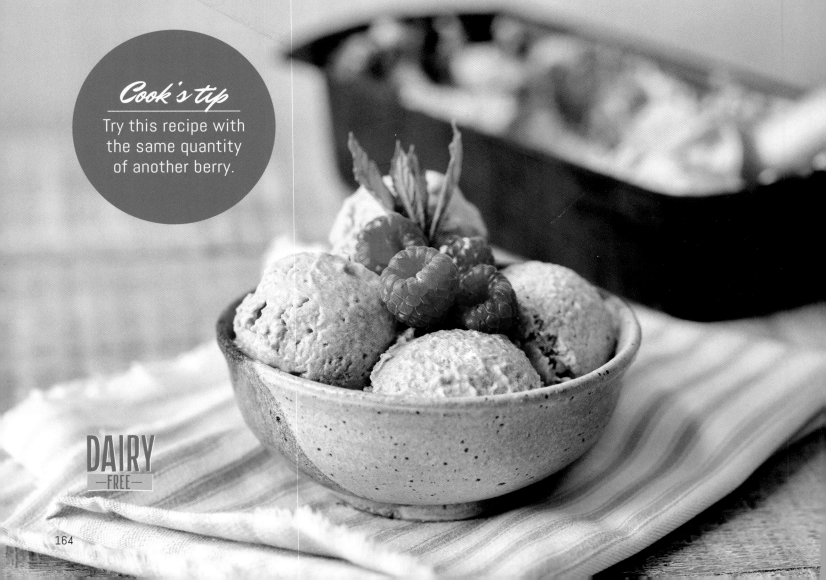